Student Workbook for
Phlebotomy
6th edition
Essent

W9-AFC-484

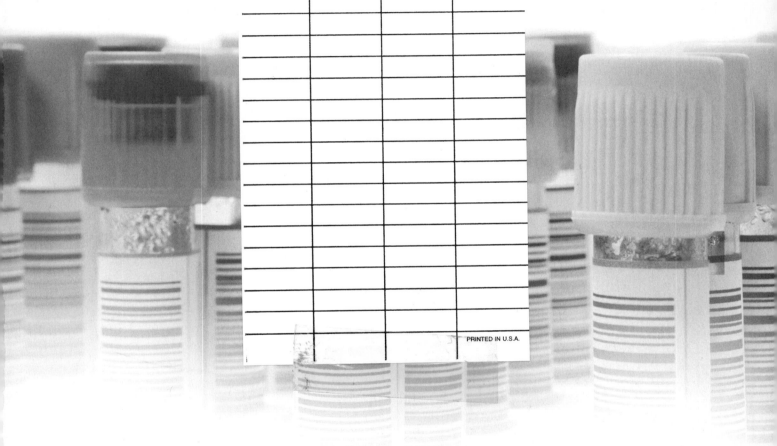

DATE DUE

NOV 3 0 2015

PRINTED IN U.S.A.

Ruth E. McCall, BS, MT (ASCP)
Retired Director of Phlebotomy and Clinical
Laboratory Assistant Programs
Central New Mexico (CNM) Community College
Albuquerque, New Mexico

Cathee M. Tankersley, BS, MT (ASCP)
President, NuHealth Educators, LLC
Faculty Emeritus
Phoenix College
Phoenix, Arizona

Wolters Kluwer

Philadelphia • Baltimore • New York • London
Buenos Aires • Hong Kong • Sydney • Tokyo

LIBRARY
MILWAUKEE AREA
TECHNICAL COLLEGE
NORTH CAMPUS
5555 West Highland Road
Mequon, Wisconsin 53092

616.0756
M122s
2016

Acquisitions Editor: Jonathan Joyce
Product Development Editor: Paula Williams
Editorial Assistant: Tish Rogers
Marketing Manager: Shauna Kelley
Production Project Manager: Marian Bellus
Design Coordinator: Terry Mallon
Artist/Illustrator: Jen Clements
Manufacturing Coordinator: Margie Orzech
Prepress Vendor: Aptara, Inc.

6th edition

© 2016 Wolters Kluwer

© 2012 Wolters Kluwer Health/Lippincott Williams & Wilkins. © 2008 Lippincott Williams & Wilkins, a Wolters Kluwer business. © 2003 Lippincott Williams & Wilkins. All rights reserved. This book is protected by copyright. No part of this book may be reproduced or transmitted in any form or by any means, including as photocopies or scanned-in or other electronic copies, or utilized by any information storage and retrieval system without written permission from the copyright owner, except for brief quotations embodied in critical articles and reviews. Materials appearing in this book prepared by individuals as part of their official duties as U.S. government employees are not covered by the above-mentioned copyright. To request permission, please contact Wolters Kluwer at Two Commerce Square, 2001 Market Street, Philadelphia, PA 19103, via email at permissions@lww.com, or via our website at lww.com (products and services).

9 8 7 6 5 4 3 2 1

Printed in the United States of America

978-1-4511-9453-1
Library of Congress Cataloging-in-Publication Data
available upon request

This work is provided "as is," and the publisher disclaims any and all warranties, express or implied, including any warranties as to accuracy, comprehensiveness, or currency of the content of this work.

This work is no substitute for individual patient assessment based upon healthcare professionals' examination of each patient and consideration of, among other things, age, weight, gender, current or prior medical conditions, medication history, laboratory data and other factors unique to the patient. The publisher does not provide medical advice or guidance and this work is merely a reference tool. Healthcare professionals, and not the publisher, are solely responsible for the use of this work including all medical judgments and for any resulting diagnosis and treatments.

Given continuous, rapid advances in medical science and health information, independent professional verification of medical diagnoses, indications, appropriate pharmaceutical selections and dosages, and treatment options should be made and healthcare professionals should consult a variety of sources. When prescribing medication, healthcare professionals are advised to consult the product information sheet (the manufacturer's package insert) accompanying each drug to verify, among other things, conditions of use, warnings and side effects and identify any changes in dosage schedule or contraindications, particularly if the medication to be administered is new, infrequently used or has a narrow therapeutic range. To the maximum extent permitted under applicable law, no responsibility is assumed by the publisher for any injury and/or damage to persons or property, as a matter of products liability, negligence law or otherwise, or from any reference to or use by any person of this work.

LWW.com

RRW0515

To all the students whom we have had the privilege of teaching and who have made our teaching careers worthwhile.

Ruth E. McCall
Cathee M. Tankersley

Reviewers

Justin Abeyta, AS
Sr Clinical Laboratory Science Instructor
Lab Sciences
Arizona Medical Training Institute
Mesa, Arizona

Diana Alagna, RN
Medical Assistant Program Director
Medical Assisting
Stone Academy
Waterbury, Connecticut

Rhonda Anderson, PBT(ASCP)ᶜᵐ
Program Manager/Phlebotomy Instructor
Corporate and Career Development, Direct Care
Phlebotomy Program
Greenville Technical College
Greenville, South Carolina

Belinda Beeman, CMA (AAMA), PBT(ASCP), MEd
Professor and Curriculum Coordinator
Medical Assisting
Goodwin College
East Hartford, Connecticut

Judith Blaney, MCLS
Phlebotomy Internship Coordinator
Allied Health
Manchester Community College
Manchester, New Hampshire

Kathy Bode, RN, BS, MS
Professor of Nursing Program
Allied Health Program Coordinator
Nursing and Allied Health
Flint Hills Technical College
Emporia, Kansas

Diane Butera, ASCP
CPT Instructor
Phlebotomy
Fortis Institute
Wayne, New Jersey

Marie Chouest, LPN
LPN Instructor
Health Sciences
Northshore Technical Community College
Bogalusa, Louisiana

Becky M. Clark, MEd, MT(ASCP)
Professor
Medical Laboratory Technology
J. Sargeant Reynolds Community College
Richmond, Virginia

Kelly Collins, MA, CPT1
Teacher
Allied Health
Tulare Adult School
Tulare, California

Silvia de la Fuente, MA, AHI
Phlebotomy Instructor
Allied Health Institute
Medical Programs and Phlebotomy
Estrella Mountain Community College
Avondale, Arizona

Desiree DeLeon, ASCP(PBT)ᶜᵐ, RN
RN Phlebotomy Instructor
Medical Lab Sciences
Central New Mexico Community
    College
Albuquerque, New Mexico

Mary Doshi, MA, MLS(ASCP)
Associate Professor/MLT Program Director
Medical Technology
San Juan College
Farmington, New Mexico

Amy Eady, MT(ASCP), MS(CTE), RMA
Director of Allied Health
Allied Health
Montcalm Community College
Sidney, Michigan

Kathleen Fowle, CPT
Certified Phlebotomist and Instructor
Pinellas Technical College
St. Joseph's Hospital
Clearwater, Florida

Tammy Gallagher, MT(ASCP)
Lead Phlebotomy Instructor
Emergency Medical Services
Butler County Community College
Butler, Pennsylvania

Faye Hamrac, MT, MS, BS
Phlebotomy Instructor
Health Sciences/Phlebotomy
Reid State Technical College
Evergreen, Alabama

Jacqueline Harris, CMA (AAMA), AHI (AMT)
Allied Health Program Chair
Medical Assisting, HCA, Medical Lab Tech
Wright Career College
Wichita, Kansas

Ronald Hedger, DO
Associate Professor of Primary Care
Clinical Education
Touro University Nevada
Henderson, Nevada

Eleanor Hooley, MT (ASCP)
Educator
Allied Health Department
Vancouver Community College
Vancouver, BC, Canada

Jamie Horn, RMA, RPT, AHI
Medical Instructor
Medical Programs
Warren County Career Center
Warren, Pennsylvania

Konnie King Briggs, CCT, CCI; PBT(ASCP); CPCI, ACA
Healthcare Instructor
Healthcare Continuing Education
Houston Community College
Houston, Texas

Theresa Kittle, CPT
Adjunct Instructor
Healthcare
Rockford Career College
Rockford, Illinois

Judy Kline, NCMA, RMA
Medical Assistant Instructor
Health Science Medical Assisting
Miami Lakes Technical Education Center
Miami Lakes, Florida

Peggy Mayo, MEd
Associate Professor
Multi-Competency Health Technology
Columbus State Community College
Columbus, Ohio

Andrea Minaya, MA, CPT
MA/CPT Lab Assistant and CPT
    Administrator
Medical Assistant and Certified Phlebotomy
    Technician
Fortis Institute
Wayne, New Jersey

Linda Pace, CMA, CPC-A
Director, Medical Assisting/Phlebotomy
Medical Assisting and Phlebotomy
Red Rocks Community College
Lakewood, Colorado

Nicole Palmieri, BSN, RN; CCMA, CPT, CET, CPCT
Instructor
Medical Assistant, Phlebotomy, Cardiac/EKG
Patient Care Technician
Advantage Career Institute
Eatontown, New Jersey

Paula Phelps, RMA
Online Education Coordinator
Allied Health
Cowley County Community College
Arkansas City, Kansas

Deyal Riley, CPT, CHI(NHA)
Instructor
Healthcare
Washtenaw Community College
Ann Arbor, Michigan

Ann Robinson, BS, MA, RPBT, LPN
Laboratory Coordinator
Phlebotomy, CNA, RMA, Surg Tech, LPN
Sports Medication
Tulsa Technology Center
Tulsa, Oklahoma

Kristie Rose, MA, PBT(ASCP), CMP
Program Manager/Instructor
Phlebotomy-Health Sciences
Eastern Florida State College
Cocoa, Florida

Diana Ross, RPT(AMT)
Career Services Coordinator
Pima Medical Institute
Mesa, Arizona

Suzanne Rouleau, MSN, RN, HHS
Educator
Allied Health
Manchester Community College
Manchester, Connecticut

Michael Simpson, BA, MS, MT(ASCP)
Clinical Laboratory Instructor
Clinical Laboratory Science
College of Southern Nevada
Clark County, Nevada

Maria V. Suto, BA, CPT
Faculty
Medical Assisting/Certified Phlebotomy Technician
Fortis Institute
Wayne, New Jersey

Joseph Tharrington, CPT1, CPT2, CPT (AMT) RPT, MA
Northern & Central Coast Regional
Director/Instructor
Phlebotomy, Medical Assisting
Academy Education Services (DBA) Clinical
   Training Institute
Santa Maria, California

Tina Veith, MA
Phlebotomy Instructor
Phlebotomy
Allied Health Careers Institute
Murfreesboro, Tennessee

Amy Vogel, MHA
Program Director, Phlebotomy Technician
Allied Health
Harrisburg Area Community College
Harrisburg, Pennsylvania

Sharon F. Whetten, MEd, BS, MT(ASCP)
Education Coordinator
TriCore Reference Laboratories
Albuquerque, New Mexico

Kari Williams, BS, DC
Director, Medical Office Technology Program
Medical Office Technology
Front Range Community College
Westminster, Colorado

Rebecca C. Wilkins, MS, MT(ASCP), SM(ASCP)
Part-time Faculty Instructor
Health Science—MLT/Phlebotomy Program
San Juan College
Farmington, New Mexico

Preface

Student Workbook for Phlebotomy Essentials, sixth edition, is designed to be used in combination with the sixth edition of the *Phlebotomy Essentials* textbook as a valuable learning resource that will help the student master the principles of phlebotomy by reinforcing key concepts and procedures covered in the textbook. The workbook offers a variety of exercises and tools to make it easy and fun for the student to understand and remember essential information and enhance critical thinking skills.

Some exercises require written answers to provide spelling practice in addition to testing knowledge. Every chapter includes:

- **Chapter Objectives** that correspond to those in the companion textbook
- **Matching Activities** including Key Term Matching using the key terms from the corresponding textbook chapter
- **Labeling Activities** to help students visualize important material
- **Knowledge Drills** including fun scrambled word activities and brand new to this edition, a True/False

activity that tests your grasp of concepts by turning a false statement into one that is true

- **Skills Drills**, including requisition and procedure practice activities
- Updated and in some cases expanded **Chapter and Unit Crossword Puzzles** to help make learning fun
- **Chapter Review Questions** to test comprehension of chapter material
- **Case Studies** to bring concepts to life including additional case studies new to this edition

Answers to all workbook activities and exercises are located in the Faculty Resource Center at http://thepoint.lww.com/McCallWorkbook6e. Access to these answers is strictly limited to faculty only. If you have further questions concerning this workbook, please email customerservice@lww.com.

The authors sincerely wish to express their gratitude to all who assisted in and supported this effort.

Ruth E. McCall
Cathee M. Tankersley

Acknowledgments

The authors would like to thank *Acquisitions Editor* **Jonathan Joyce** and the production and editorial staff at Wolters Kluwer, especially those with whom we worked most closely, with a special thank you to *Product Development Editor* **Paula Williams**, *Creative Services Art Director* **Jennifer Clements** and *Supervisor of Product Development* **Eve Malakoff-Klein** for their patience, support, and dedication to this endeavor, and an extra special thank you to Eve for stepping in and taking the lead when it was really needed. We also wish to give special recognition to our compositor **Indu Jawwad** and her team at Aptara for their patience and professionalism as they brought together the many components of all three texts.

Contents

Chapter 1

Phlebotomy: Past and Present and the Healthcare Setting

Objectives

Study the information in your TEXTBOOK that corresponds to each objective to prepare yourself for the activities in this chapter.

1 Demonstrate basic knowledge of terminology for healthcare settings including the national healthcare organizations that contributed to the evolution of phlebotomy and the role of the phlebotomist today.

2 Describe the basic concepts of verbal and nonverbal communication as they relate to the professional image and proper telephone protocol in the health care.

3 Compare types of healthcare institutions and the methods used by providers for coverage.

4 List the personnel levels in the clinical analysis areas of the laboratory and the types of laboratory procedures performed in each of the areas.

Matching

Use choices only once unless otherwise indicated.

MATCHING 1-1: KEY TERMS AND DESCRIPTIONS

Match the key term with the *best* description.

Key Terms (1–16)

1. _____ ACA
2. _____ ACO
3. _____ AHCCCS
4. _____ certification
5. _____ CLIA '88
6. _____ communication barriers
7. _____ CMS
8. _____ CPT
9. _____ case manager
10. _____ exsanguinate
11. _____ HIPAA
12. _____ HMOs
13. _____ ICD-10-PCS
14. _____ IDN
15. _____ kinesic slip
16. _____ kinesics

Descriptions

A. Evidence that an individual has mastered fundamental competencies in a technical specialty
B. Health Insurance Portability and Accountability Act
C. Accountable Care Organization
D. Experienced HC professional who serves as the patient's advocate and adviser
E. Verbal and nonverbal messages do not match
F. Health maintenance organizations
G. Arizona Health Care Cost Containment System
H. Current procedural terminology codes
I. Biases that are major obstructions to verbal communication
J. *International Classification of Diseases,* 10th Revision
K. Clinical Laboratory Improvement Amendments of 1988
L. Patient Protection and Affordable Care Act
M. Centers for Medicare and Medicaid Services
N. Integrated delivery network
O. Study of nonverbal communication
P. Remove or drain all blood

Key Terms (17–32)

17. _____ MCO
18. _____ Medicaid
19. _____ Medicare
20. _____ MLS
21. _____ PCP
22. _____ PHI
23. _____ PHS
24. _____ phlebotomy
25. _____ polycythemia
26. _____ PM
27. _____ primary care
28. _____ proxemics
29. _____ reference laboratories
30. _____ secondary care
31. _____ tertiary care
32. _____ third-party payer

Descriptions

A. Care by physician who assumes ongoing responsibility for maintaining patients' health.
B. Care by specialist who can perform out-of-the-ordinary procedures in outpatient facilities
C. More recent term meaning venesection
D. Disorder involving overproduction of red blood cells
E. Highly complex care from practitioners in a hospital or overnight facility
F. Managed care organization
G. Federally funded program that provides health care to seniors, 65 and older
H. Primary Care Physician
I. Promotes and administers programs for public health
J. Federal and state program that provides medical assistance for eligible low-income Americans
K. Insurance company that pays for healthcare services on behalf of a patient
L. Personalized medicine
M. Study of an individual's concept and use of space
N. Large, independent laboratories that test specimens from many different facilities
O. Medical Laboratory Scientist
P. Protected health information

MATCHING 1-2: CERTIFICATION AGENCIES

Match the certification agency with the title awarded. *A title may be used more than once.*

Certification Agency

1. _____ American Society of Clinical Pathologists

2. _____ American Medical Technologists

3. _____ National Center for Competency Testing

4. _____ American Certification Agency

Title Awarded

A. RPT
B. CPT
C. PBT
D. NCPT

MATCHING 1-3: METHODS OF PAYMENT AND DIAGNOSIS CODING

Match the methods of payment and diagnosis coding with the appropriate definition.

Method of Payment and Diagnosis Coding

1. _____ Ambulatory patient classification

2. _____ *International Classification of Diseases,* 10th Revision

3. _____ Fee for Service

4. _____ Diagnosis-related groups

5. _____ Prospective Payment System

Definitions

A. Begun in 1983 to limit and standardize the Medicare/ Medicaid payments made to hospitals
B. Reimburses healthcare facilities a set amount for each patient procedure using established disease categories
C. A classification system implemented in 2000 for determining payment to healthcare facilities for Medicare and Medicaid patients only
D. Traditional payment model of reimbursement for healthcare service after service is rendered
E. A procedural classification system for use in U.S. hospitals with a broad range of codes and greater specificity

MATCHING 1-4: LABORATORY TESTS AND DEPARTMENTS

Match the laboratory tests with the departments that perform them. *Departments can be used more than one time.*

Laboratory Tests

1. _____ BUN

2. _____ PT

3. _____ Hct

4. _____ WBC diff

5. _____ Nitrites

6. _____ ANA

7. _____ Fibrinogen

8. _____ ALT

9. _____ D-dimer

10. _____ Pap smear

11. _____ Blood culture

12. _____ EBV

13. _____ Type and Rh

14. _____ Gram stain

15. _____ DAT

16. _____ Immunoglobulins

17. _____ Creatinine

18. _____ APTT

19. _____ Plt ct

20. _____ hsCRP

21. _____ pH

22. _____ Occult blood

23. _____ Urobilinogen

24. _____ Potassium

Laboratory Departments

A. Hematology
B. Blood Bank
C. Coagulation
D. Chemistry
E. Immunology
F. Urinalysis
G. Microbiology
H. Cytology

MATCHING 1-5: PATIENT CONDITIONS AND MEDICAL SPECIALTIES

Match the specialties with types of patient conditions they serve.

Patient Conditions

1. _____ Tumors, benign and malignant

2. _____ Eye examinations

3. _____ Endocrine gland disorders

4. _____ Diseases of the heart

5. _____ Disorders of the brain and spinal cord

6. _____ Well checkups for children

7. _____ Kidney function

8. _____ Urinary tract disease

9. _____ Conditions of the skin

10. _____ Emergent care due to accident

11. _____ Injuries resulting from athletic activities

12. _____ Respiratory system conditions

13. _____ Inflammation and joint diseases

14. _____ Contagious, pathogenic infections

15. _____ Disorders of the blood

16. _____ Disorders causing hypersensitivity

17. _____ Age-related disorders

18. _____ Clinical depression

19. _____ Digestive tract disorders

20. _____ Continuous, comprehensive care

Medical Specialties

A. Allergy & Immunology

B. Anesthesiology

C. Cardiology

D. Dermatology

E. Emergency Medicine

F. Endocrinology

G. Family Medicine

H. Gastroenterology

I. Gerontology

J. Hematology

K. Infectious Diseases

L. Nephrology

M. Neurology

N. Oncology

O. Ophthalmology

P. Pediatrics

Q. Psychiatry

R. Pulmonary Medicine

S. Rheumatology

T. Sports Medicine

Labeling Exercises

LABELING EXERCISE 1-1: VERBAL COMMUNICATION BARRIERS

Using the TEXTBOOK, identify six barriers in the communication loop diagram that interrupt the message being sent to the receiver. Write the answers in the Receiver's column. Identify six communication barriers that interrupt the feedback being sent to the sender. Write the answers in the Sender's column.

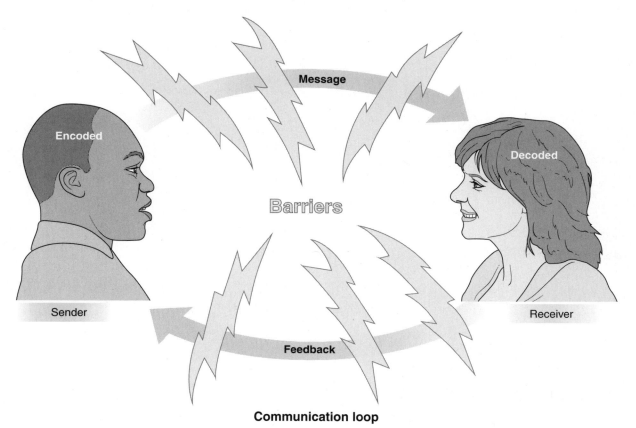

Communication loop

Receiver	Sender
1. _____	1. _____
2. _____	2. _____
3. _____	3. _____
4. _____	4. _____
5. _____	5. _____
6. _____	6. _____

LABELING EXERCISE 1-2: NONVERBAL FACIAL CUES

Label each of the sketches below with the correct facial cue from the following list. Answers may be used more than once.

- Surprise
- Fear
- Sad
- Happy
- Anger
- Disgust

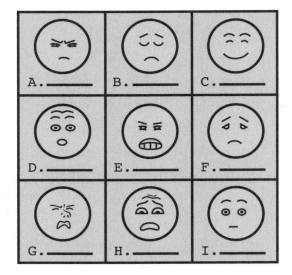

LABELING EXERCISE 1-3: LABORATORY ORGANIZATIONAL CHART

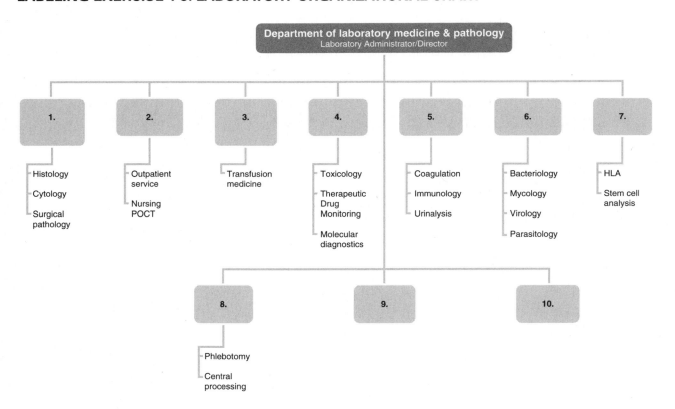

Fill in the names of the major divisions in a typical laboratory organizational chart.

1. _____

2. _____

3. _____

4. _____

5. _____

6. _____

7. _____

8. _____

9. _____

10. _____

Knowledge Drills

KNOWLEDGE DRILL 1-1: CAUTION AND KEY POINT RECOGNITION

The following sentences have been taken from caution and key point statements found throughout Chapter 1 of the textbook. Using the TEXTBOOK, fill in the blanks with the missing information.

1. By recognizing and appreciating (A) _____, the phlebotomist promotes (B) _____ and harmonious relationships that directly improve health (C) _____, the (D) _____ of services, and (E) _____ satisfaction.

2. The (A) _____ phrase *primum non nocere*, which means "first do no harm" describes one of the fundamental (B) _____ of health care. Although it does not include this (C) _____ _____, the promise "to abstain from doing harm" is part of the (D) _____ oath given to new physicians and other (E) _____ professionals as they begin their practice.

3. To (A) _____ effectively with someone, it is important to establish good (B) _____ _____. A patient or client may be made to feel (C) _____ and more like an (D) _____ rather than a human being if no eye contact is established.

4. Phlebotomists will find that when dealing with (A) _____ who are (B) _____ or (C) _____, a confident and professional (D) _____ will be most (E) _____ to them in doing their job.

5. An important (A) _____ in ensuring that the healthcare system as a whole is (B) _____ is the (C) _____ _____ physician (PCP). It has been shown that (D) _____ primary care results in better health outcomes and lower spending, including avoidable (E) _____ _____ visits and hospital care.

KNOWLEDGE DRILL 1-2: SCRAMBLED WORDS

Unscramble the following words using the hints given in parenthesis and the letters that have been placed in the correct boxes. Finish writing the correct spelling of the scrambled word in the corresponding box.

1. deadmici _____ (health care for the poor)

		d				i	

2. enscikis _____ (involves body language)

	i			s			

3. fracitinecito _____ (an indication of competency)

C				i						i		

4. gloomyheat _____ (lab area that counts blood cells)

		m				l			

5. irebrar _____ (message obstruction)

		r				r	

6. mexicrops _____ (involves one's concept of space)

		o		m			

7. ratyitre _____ (highly complex care)

						r	y	

8. shymictre _____ (most lab tests are this type)

		e	m					

9. sneeviconte _____ (phlebotomy)

V										n	

10. troblumaya _____ (describes most outpatients)

		b			a				

KNOWLEDGE DRILL 1-3: TRUE/FALSE

The following statements are all false. Circle the one or two words that make the statement false and write the correct word(s) that would make the statement true in the space provided.

1. One CEU equals 20 contact hours of participation in an organized experience under responsible sponsorship, capable direction, and qualified instruction.

2. A continued awareness and knowledge of cultural differences by all employees can protect an organization from OSHA and HIPAA violations, promote an inviting workplace, and increase innovation and teamwork.

3. Ethics are centered on an individual's emotions.

4. All patients in a healthcare setting have rights but do not have to be informed of these rights when care is initiated.

5. Safeguarding the correctness of protected health information (PHI) is one of the primary aims of the Joint Commission's privacy rule.

6. The Latin phrase *primum non nocere*, which means "do not ignore the patient" describes one of the fundamental principles of health care.

7. Most phlebotomists' work is in the personal zone as they search and palpate to find a vein and perform venipuncture.

8. Today, assisted living centers are seen as a way to decrease the overcrowded emergency rooms and provide significant savings to patients and insurers.

9. An important component in ensuring that the healthcare system as a whole is sustainable is the specialist physician.

10. Certification is a required process by which a hospital grants recognition to an individual who has met certain prerequisites in a particular technical area.

KNOWLEDGE DRILL 1-4: HISTORICAL PHLEBOTOMY EVENTS

Number the following events in chronological order from 1 to 5, with 1 being the earliest recorded event.

a. _____ The French used leeching for localized bloodletting.

b. _____ "Short robe" surgeons used cupping and leeching to extract blood.

c. _____ Microsurgeons use leeching to lessen the complications of surgery.

d. _____ Hippocrates used bloodletting to cleanse the body of impurities.

e. _____ Physicians used a procedure called venesection to treat George Washington.

KNOWLEDGE DRILL 1-5: INPATIENT/OUTPATIENT FACILITY

Write the correct category (outpatient or inpatient) of healthcare facility in the line provided before the statement description.

1. _____ Principal source of healthcare services for most people

2. _____ Highly complex services

3. _____ Requires that patients stay overnight or longer

4. _____ Center of the American healthcare system

5. _____ Same-day surgical procedures

6. _____ Physician's office care

KNOWLEDGE DRILL 1-6: MEDICARE/MEDICAID PROGRAMS

Write the correct program name (Medicare or Medicaid) in the line provided before the statement description.

1. _____ Funds come from federal grants

2. _____ An entitlement program

3. _____ Provides medical assistance to the poor

4. _____ Program administered by the state

5. _____ Benefits divided into two sections: Part A and Part B

6. _____ Financed through social security deductions

KNOWLEDGE DRILL 1-7: PROFESSIONAL ATTITUDE

After each characteristic listed below, define and describe how this quality contributes to your professional attitude:

a. Self-confidence _____

_____

_____

b. Self-motivation _____

_____

_____

c. Compassion _____

_____

_____

d. Dependability _____

_____

_____

e. Ethical behavior _____

_____

_____

f. Integrity _____

_____

_____

Skills Drills

SKILLS DRILL 1-1: REQUISITION ACTIVITY

Instructions: A test requisition contains the following test abbreviations. Write the complete name of the test and the department that will perform the test on the corresponding line next to the abbreviation.

Any Hospital USA
1123 West Physician Drive
Any Town USA

Laboratory Test Requisition

- -

PATIENT INFORMATION:

Name: _____ Smith _____ Jane _____ R _____
          (last)   (first)   (MI)

Identification Number: __09365784__   Birth Date: _06/21/63_

Referring Physician: __Coleman__

Date to be Collected: __08/11/15__   Time to be Collected: __0600__

Special Instructions: __line draw only__

- -

TEST(S) REQUIRED:

TEST ABBREVIATION	TEST NAME	DEPARTMENT
1. RBC		
2. Hgb		
3. FDP		
4. BUN		
5. PT		
6. CBC		
7. AST		
8. RF		
9. UA		
10. C&S		

SKILLS DRILL 1-2: WORD BUILDING (See Chapter 4, Medical Terminology)

Divide each of the words below into all of its elements (parts): prefix (P), word root (WR), combining vowel (CV), and suffix (S). Write the word part and its definition on the corresponding lines. Write the general meaning of the word in the space provided. If the word does not have a particular element, write NA (not applicable) in its place.

Example: pathology

Elements _____ /_____*path*_____ /_____*o*_____ /_____*logy*_____
                    P   WR   CV   S

Definitions _____ /_____*disease*_____ /_____ /_____*study of*_____

Meaning: study of disease

1. nephrology

   Elements _____ /_____ /_____ /_____
                  P   WR   CV   S

   Definition _____ /_____ /_____ /_____

   Meaning:

2. phlebotomy

   Elements _____ /_____ /_____ /_____
                  P   WR   CV   S

   Definition _____ /_____ /_____ /_____

   Meaning:

3. polycythemia

   Elements _____ /_____ /_____ /_____ /_____
                  P   WR   CV   WR   S

   Definition _____ /_____ /_____ /_____ /_____

   Meaning:

4. hematology

   Elements _____ /_____ /_____ /_____
                  P   WR   CV   S

   Definition _____ /_____ /_____ /_____

   Meaning:

5. erythrocyte

   Elements _____ /_____ /_____ /_____
                  P   WR   CV   S

   Definition _____ /_____ /_____ /_____

   Meaning:

6. dermatologist

   Elements _____ /_____ /_____ /_____
                  P   WR   CV   S

   Definition _____ /_____ /_____ /_____

   Meaning:

SKILLS DRILL 1-3: PROPER TELEPHONE ETIQUETTE

Fill in the blanks of the following table with the missing information.

Proper Etiquette	Communication Tips	Rationale
Answer (1) _____.		• If the phone is allowed to ring too many times, the caller may assume that the people working in the laboratory are inefficient or (2) _____.
State your name and department.		• The caller has the right to know to whom he or she is speaking.
Be helpful.	Ask how you can be of help to the (3) _____ and facilitate the conversation. Keep your statements and answers simple and to the point so as to avoid confusion.	• When a phone rings, it is because someone needs something. Because of the nature of the healthcare business, the caller may be (4) _____ and may benefit from hearing a calm, pleasant voice at the other end.
(5) _____ calls.	Inform a caller if he or she is interrupting a call from someone else. Always ask permission before putting a caller on hold in case it is an (8) _____ that must be handled immediately.	• It takes an (6) _____ person to coordinate several calls. Being able to triage is an important (7) _____ that takes a knowledgeable and experienced person to handle well. • The caller needs to know where they are in the queue. Handling an important call or an emergency (9) _____ will save the laboratory from problems in the future.
Transfer and put (10) _____ properly.	Tell a caller when you are going to transfer the call or put it on hold and learn how to do this in the right way. **Note:** Do not leave the line open and do not keep the caller waiting too long.	• Disconnecting callers while transferring or putting them on hold (11) _____ them. • Leaving the line open, so that other conversations can be heard by the person on hold is discourteous and can compromise (12) _____. • (13) _____ back with a caller when on hold for longer than expected; this keeps him or her informed of the circumstance. • If a caller is waiting on hold too long, ask if he or she would like to leave a (14) _____.

Be prepared to record information.

Have a pencil and paper close to the phone.

- Listen (15) _____, which means clarifying, (17) _____, and summarizing the information received.

- Documentation is necessary when answering the phone at work to ensure that (16) _____ information is transmitted to the necessary person.

- Reading back the information when complete is one of best ways to (18) _____ it is correct.

Know the laboratory's policies.

Make answers consistent by learning the laboratory's policies.

- People who answer the telephone must know the laboratory (19) _____ to avoid giving the wrong information. Misinformation given to the caller can result in unnecessary worry and additional expense.

- (20) _____ answers help establish the laboratory's credibility because a caller's perception of the lab involves more than just accurate test results.

Defuse (21) _____ situations.

When a caller is hostile, you might say "I can see why you are upset. Let me see what I can do."

- Some callers become angry because of lost results or errors in billing.

- (22) _____ a hostile caller's (23) _____ will often defuse the situation.

- After the caller has calmed down, the issue can be addressed.

Try to assist everyone.

If you are uncertain, refer the caller to someone who can address the caller's issue.

Remind yourself to keep your attention on (25) _____ _____ at a time.

- It is possible to assist callers and (24) _____ _____ even if you are not actually answering their questions.

- Validate callers' requests by giving a response that tells them something (26)_____ _____ done.

- (27) _____ interest in the caller will enhance communication and contribute to the good (28) _____ of the laboratory.

SKILLS DRILL 1-4: TWO CATEGORIES OF HEALTHCARE FACILITIES

Outpatient

- (1) _____ source of healthcare services for most people.

- Offer (3) _____ care in physician's office to (4) _____ care in a freestanding ambulatory setting.

- Serve (5) _____ care physicians who assume (7) _____ responsibility for maintaining patients' health.

- Serve (8) _____ care physicians (specialists) who perform routine surgery, (10) _____ treatments, therapeutic radiology, and so on in same-day service centers.

Inpatient

- The key resource and (2) _____ of the American healthcare system.

- Offer specialized instrumentation and technology to assist in unusual diagnoses and treatments.

- Serve (6) _____ care (highly complex services and therapy) practitioners. Usually requires that patients stay overnight or longer.

- Examples are acute care hospitals, nursing homes, (9) _____ care facilities, (11) _____, and (12) _____ centers.

Crossword

ACROSS

1. Federal healthcare program for persons 65 years of age and older
6. Occupational Safety & Health Administration (abbrev.)
8. Personalized filters or biases
10. Internationally recognized standard formula for PT results
11. Electroencephalogram (abbrev.)
12. Protected health information (abbrev.)
14. State of being varied or different
17. Cervical smear for cancer cells
18. Complete blood counts (abbrev.)
19. Continuing education unit (abbrev.)
20. Center for Medicare and Medicaid (abbrev.)
22. Identifying with the feelings of another person
23. Therapeutic _____, nonverbal communication
26. Prepaid managed care group practices
27. Disseminated intravascular coagulation (abbrev.)
29. Intensive care unit (abbrev.)
31. Coagulation test used to detect heparin
33. Arizona's version of Medicaid
35. Hemoglobin (abbrev.)
36. Urinalysis (abbrev.)
37. "Blood _____" to rid body of evil spirits
39. Health maintenance organization (abbrev.)
40. Word meaning "immediate"
42. Emotion brought on by feeling out of control
43. Alanine aminotransferase (abbrev.)

DOWN

1. Hemoglobin concentration in RBCs (abbrev.)
2. Standard or requirement for a technical specialty
3. Registered nurses (abbrev.)
4. Wrongful act committed against one's person
5. Study of nonverbal communication
7. Condition of decreased RBCs in blood
8. Basic metabolic panel (abbrev.)
9. Standards of right or wrong conduct
13. Federal HC program for the indigent
15. Unquestioning belief in the HCW's ability
16. _____ stain for bacteria
21. American Hospital Association (abbrev.)
22. Complete removal of all blood
24. Occupation therapy (abbrev.)
25. Organization that offers continuing education
26. Federal law that protects patient confidentiality
28. Personal standard of honesty
30. _____ medicinalis
32. Stool sample may show this stage of a parasite
34. To confirm specific qualifications have been met
37. Laboratory information system (abbrev.)
38. Phlebotomy certifying agency that united with ASCP
39. Hematocrit (abbrev.)
41. Turnaround time (abbrev.)

Chapter Review Questions

1. In the 17th century, the name given to the blood-letting tool or lancet was
   - a. cup.
   - b. fleam.
   - c. hemostat.
   - d. leech.

2. A factor that contributes to the overall professional impression made by the phlebotomist is
   - a. compassion.
   - b. dependability.
   - c. self-confidence.
   - d. any of the above.

3. After successful completion of the American Medical Technologists phlebotomy examination, the initials for the title granted are
   - a. CPT.
   - b. CLT.
   - c. PBT.
   - d. RPT.

4. Understanding the _____ of a diverse population is very important in providing health care.
   - a. history
   - b. motivation
   - c. traditions
   - d. all the above

5. The evidence that an individual has mastered fundamental competencies in his or her technical area is called
   - a. certification.
   - b. ethics.
   - c. esteem.
   - d. tort.

6. Developed by AMA to provide a terminology and coding system for physician billing
   - a. APC
   - b. CPT
   - c. DRG
   - d. Medicare

7. Which of the following is the responsibility of a phlebotomist?
   - a. Analyze specimens
   - b. Dispatch samples
   - c. Obtain vital signs
   - d. Transport patients

8. Which of the following is an example of proxemics?
   - a. Eye contact
   - b. Zone of comfort
   - c. Facial expressions
   - d. Personal hygiene

9. Which of the following is improper telephone technique?
   - a. Listening and restating information
   - b. Putting an irritated caller on hold
   - c. Taking notes as the caller is talking
   - d. Referring the caller elsewhere if uncertain

10. A healthcare facility that provides ambulatory services is a/an
    - a. acute-care hospital.
    - b. assisted living home.
    - c. rehabilitation center.
    - d. urgent care center.

11. The name of a federal entitlement program is
    - a. IDN.
    - b. HIPPA.
    - c. managed care.
    - d. Medicare.

12. The specialty that treats disorders of the brain is called
    - a. cardiology.
    - b. gerontology.
    - c. neurology.
    - d. pathology.

13. The department in the hospital that treats lung deficiencies is
    - a. clinical laboratory.
    - b. diagnostic imaging.
    - c. electroneurodiagnostics.
    - d. respiratory therapy.

14. The histology department in the laboratory performs
    - a. blood culture testing.
    - b. compatibility testing.
    - c. electrolyte monitoring.
    - d. tissue processing.

15. The abbreviation for the serology test that indicates the presence of Hepatitis C is called
    - a. AST.
    - b. CMV.
    - c. FSP.
    - d. HCV.

16. Which of the following laboratory professionals is specified by CLIA as responsible for evaluating new procedures?
    - a. Laboratory manager
    - b. Medical laboratory scientist
    - c. Medical laboratory technician
    - d. Technical supervisor

17. An important component in ensuring that the healthcare system is sustainable in the future is the
    - a. administration of drug abuse programs.
    - b. consistent use of primary care physicians.
    - c. elimination of ambulatory services.
    - d. increased use of emergency medicine.

18. Some managed care attempts to control costs by
    a. allowing patients to choose their own providers.
    b. discouraging preventative medicine.
    c. permitting patient unlimited healthcare service.
    d. using case managers to monitor patients.

19. The healthcare reform bill, better known as ACA is
    a. designed to reform the insurance market.
    b. eliminating managed care options.
    c. reduce access to tertiary care facilities.
    d. increase Public Health Services clinics.

20. Healthcare providers who do not recognize diversity are
    a. increasing innovation and teamwork.
    b. promoting interpersonal relations.
    c. risking a civil right's violation.
    d. supporting greater job satisfaction.

Case Studies

Case Study 1-1: More Education for the OJT Phlebotomist

The phlebotomist, Sam, has been trained on the job (OJT) and since that is how everyone else currently in the physician's office was trained, he doesn't see it as a problem. One thing bothers him, however, and it is that no one seems to be able to answer questions that come up daily about the rationale for doing phlebotomy procedures a certain way. The answer is always the same: "I don't know. It has always been done that way." When the physician's office was notified of a pending visit from CLIA inspectors, it was decided that all the phlebotomists should get credentials, if possible, and in that way every phlebotomist would better understand his or her job responsibilities.

QUESTIONS

1. What does "getting credentialed" mean as far as phlebotomists are concerned?

2. How can Sam become officially recognized as a phlebotomist?

3. Where can Sam go to receive a standardized educational curriculum that incorporates classroom instruction and clinical practice in phlebotomy?

4. How can Sam keep current after he becomes credentialed?

Case Study 1-2: Nonverbal Cues Speak Loudly

The patient did not understand English, but this was not unusual in the County Hospital. Donna, the phlebotomist, spoke only English and could not tell the patient why she was there or what was going to happen. She had learned that the best way to handle this situation was to continue preparing her equipment, nodding her head often to affirm the patient's comments but never really looking the patient in the eye. This particular time the patient continued to talk nervously and did not offer his arm. As Donna glanced up to see why he hadn't, she saw an intense frown on his face and that his eyes were narrowed. His hand was actually clenched, and he was leaning back in his bed as far as he could. Donna proceeded by grasping his arm and forcefully moving it toward her. She quickly tied the tourniquet, cleaned the area, and prepared to stick the median cubital vein. Just as she got the needle through the skin, the patient yelled and pulled the needle out of his arm.

QUESTIONS

1. What did Donna's nonverbal cues say to the patient?

2. What nonverbal signals were the patient offering to Donna?

3. What should the facial and hand cues from the patient have told Donna?

4. How could this situation have been handled differently?

Case Study 1-3: Understanding Healthcare Reform

A patient arrives at her doctor's office for an annual complete exam. Upon arrival, she finds that the doctor has just recently joined an ACO. The patient is immediately suspicious of the system, thinking it sounds like an HMO, something she does not like. At the end of the visit, she is given a requisition for blood work to be done by the laboratory of an ACO-affiliated hospital. The patient does not really like that hospital and chooses to go somewhere else.

QUESTIONS

1. What do the letters ACA and ACO stand for?

2. What role does the ACA play in this physician's decision to be in an ACO?

3. Why would a physician join an ACO?

4. Is an ACO another name for HMO?

5. Has the patient violated the physician's orders by going to another lab?

Chapter 2

Quality Assurance and Legal Issues in Healthcare

Objectives

Study the information in your TEXTBOOK that corresponds to each objective to prepare yourself for the activities in this chapter.

1 Demonstrate basic knowledge of terminology for national organizations, agencies, and regulations that support quality assurance in health care.

2 Define quality and performance improvement measurements as they relate to phlebotomy, and describe the components of a quality assurance (QA) program and identify areas in phlebotomy subject to quality control (QC).

3 Demonstrate knowledge of the legal aspects associated with phlebotomy procedures by defining legal terminology and describing situations that may have legal ramifications.

Matching

Use choices only once unless otherwise indicated.

MATCHING 2-1: KEY TERMS AND DESCRIPTIONS

Match each key term with the *best* description.

Key Terms (1–16)

1. _____ Assault
2. _____ Battery
3. _____ Breach of confidentiality
4. _____ Civil action
5. _____ CLSI
6. _____ CMS
7. _____ CQI
8. _____ Defendant
9. _____ Delta check
10. _____ Deposition
11. _____ Discovery
12. _____ Due care
13. _____ Fraud
14. _____ GLPs
15. _____ IQCP
16. _____ Informed consent

Descriptions

A. Program designed for continuous self-evaluation and process improvement
B. Federal agency that administers the CLIA
C. Develops voluntary standards and guidelines for the laboratory
D. Current laboratory test results compared with previous test results on the same patient
E. False portrayal of facts either by words or by conduct
F. New addition to CLIA quality control policies
G. Failure to keep privileged medical information private
H. Formal process in litigation that involves taking depositions and interrogating parties involved
I. Practices that emphasize QA in all laboratory setting
J. Implies voluntary and competent permission for a medical test or procedure
K. Intentional offensive touching or use of force without consent or legal justification
L. Legal actions in which the alleged injured party sues for monetary damages
M. Level of care a sensible person provides under given circumstances
N. Person against whom a complaint is filed
O. One party questions another under oath with a court reporter present
P. Act or threat causing another to be in fear of immediate battery

Key Terms (17–32)

17. _____ Invasion of privacy
18. _____ Malpractice
19. _____ Negligence
20. _____ PSC
21. _____ NPSGs
22. _____ Plaintiff
23. _____ QA
24. _____ QC
25. _____ Quality indicators
26. _____ *Respondeat superior*
27. _____ Standard of care
28. _____ TJC
29. _____ Statute of limitations
30. _____ Threshold values
31. _____ Tort
32. _____ Vicarious liability

Descriptions

A. Accredits and certifies 20,000 health care organizations.
B. Guides used to monitor all areas of patient care
C. Injured party in the litigation process
D. Latin phrase meaning "let the master respond"
E. Length of time after alleged injury in which a lawsuit can be filed
F. Level of acceptable practice beyond which quality cannot be assured
G. Liability imposed on one person for acts committed by another
H. Small outpatient phlebotomy service center
I. A form of procedural control used to detect problems that occur
J. A component of a CQI program that is required for TJC accreditation
K. Type of negligence implying a greater standard of care was due the injured person
L. Program to prevent problems by evaluating present and past performances
M. Failure to exercise due care
N. Violation of one's right to be left alone
O. Wrongful act committed against one's person, property, or reputation
P. Level of skill that provides due care for patients

MATCHING 2-2: TYPE OF CONSENT

Type of Consent

1. _____ Informed consent

2. _____ Expressed consent

3. _____ Implied consent

4. _____ HIV consent

5. _____ Minor consent

6. _____ Refusal of consent

Description

A. A constitutional right to decline a medical procedure

B. Consent is suggested by actions

C. Implies voluntary and competent permission

D. Parental/guardian consent required for medical treatment

E. Required before surgery or high-risk procedures

F. State laws specify the information that must be given

MATCHING 2-3: NATIONAL STANDARD AND REGULATORY AGENCIES

Match the organizations and regulatory agencies to the service they provide to the laboratory community.

Organizations and Regulatory Agencies

A. CAP
B. CLIA
C. CLSI
D. NAACLS
E. TJC

Services Provided

1. _____ Developed NPSGs as an overall CQI requirement for accreditation

2. _____ Federal regulations establishing quality standards for all laboratories including physicians' offices

3. _____ Accredits and certifies health care organization and programs throughout the United States

4. _____ CLIAC was formed to assist in administering these regulations

5. _____ Develops voluntary guidelines and standards for all areas of the laboratory

6. _____ An authority on quality clinical laboratory education

7. _____ An exclusively pathologists' organization that inspects and accredits laboratories

8. _____ Developed sentinel event policy for patient safety in health care settings

9. _____ Performs external peer reviews for accreditation and approval of laboratory programs

10. _____ Inspects and accredits laboratories other than The Joint Commission

Labeling Exercises

LABELING EXERCISE 2-1: MICROBIOLOGY QUALITY ASSESSMENT FORM (Text Fig. 2-1)

Answers to the following questions can be found on the Quality Assessment and Improvement Tracking form below. Circle the answer on the form; write the number of the question in or near the circle; then write out the answer on the appropriate line.

HOSPITAL & HEALTH CENTER
QUALITY ASSESSMENT AND IMPROVEMENT TRACKING
CONFIDENTIAL A.R.S. 36-445 et. seq.

STANDARD OF CARE/SERVICE:

IMPORTANT ASPECT OF CARE/SERVICE:
LABORATORY SERVICES
COLLECTION/TRANSPORT

SIGNATURES:

_____
DIRECTOR

_____
MEDICAL DIRECTOR

_____
VICE PRESIDENT/ADMINISTRATOR

DEPARTMENTS:
DATA SOURCE(S):
METHODOLOGY: [X] RETROSPECTIVE [   ] CONCURRENT
TYPE: [   ] STRUCTURE [   ] PROCESS [X] OUTCOME
PERSON RESPONSIBLE FOR:
• DATA COLLECTION: J. HERRIG
• DATA ORGANIZATION: J. HERRIG
• ACTION PLAN: J. HERRIG
• FOLLOW-UP: J. HERRIG
DATE MONITORING BEGAN: 1990
TIME PERIOD THIS MONITOR: 2ND QUARTER 2009
MONITOR DISCONTINUED BECAUSE:
FOLLOW-UP:

INDICATORS	THLD	ACT	PREV	CRITICAL ANALYSIS/EVALUATION	ACTION PLAN
Blood Culture contamination rate will not exceed 3%				**Population: All patients** All monthly indicators were under threshold, 3%	**Share results and analysis with Lab staff and ER staff.**
APR - # of Draws: 713 　　# Contaminated: 13	3.00%	1.8%	1.2%	% Contamination from draws other than Line draws, by unit:	
MAY - # of Draws: 710 　　# Contaminated: 23	3.00%	2.8%	2.3%	APR: ER =　4.7%　Lab = 0.7% MAY: ER = 11.5%　Lab = 1.0% JUN: ER =　8.6%　Lab = 1.1%	
JUN - # of Draws: 702 　　# Contaminated: 17	3.00%	2.4%	1.9%	ER was over threshold for each month of quarter.	
Total for 1st Quarter - 　　# of Draws: 2125 　　# Contaminated: 50	3.00%	2.4%	1.9%		

---

1. What is being used by the Microbiology Department as a blood culture quality indicator? _____

2. What is the acceptable threshold? _____

3. What was the actual percentage contamination for the first quarter? _____

4. Which month has the highest contamination from ER draws? _____

5. What was the rate of contamination by the laboratory in the same month? _____

6. What is the action plan for blood culture QA? _____

LABELING 2-2: REFERENCE MANUAL (Text Fig. 2-4)

Describe what each numbered item on the underlined portion of the reference manual page (Text Fig. 2-4) tells the reader about the lab test. Write the answer on the corresponding line below.

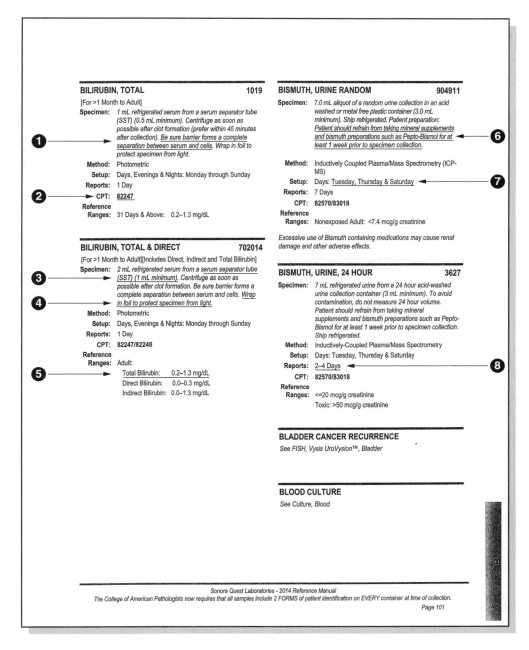

1. Specimen processing precautions
   _____

2. _____

3. _____

4. _____

5. _____

6. _____

7. _____

8. _____

Knowledge Drills

KNOWLEDGE DRILL 2-1: CAUTION AND KEY POINT RECOGNITION

The following sentences are taken from "CAUTION and KEY POINT" statements found throughout Chapter 2 in the TEXTBOOK. Using the TEXTBOOK, fill in the blanks with the missing information.

1. A person doing phlebotomy must use at least (A) _____ identifiers for patient

   (B) _____. The patient's room number or physical location (C) _____ be used as an

   identifier. For (D) _____ without ID bands, the agency requirements are met when the patient's

   (E)_____ name is compared with the name on the requisition and the patient provides a

   (F) _____ verbal identifier such as (G) _____ date or phone number.

2. There have been cases where patient (A) _____ on computer labels was (B) _____

   because incorrect information had been entered into the computer upon patient (C) _____.

   (D) _____ patient ID procedures can catch such errors.

3. For (A) _____ reasons, access to a patient's medical record is (B) _____ to

   those who have a verifiable (C) _____ to review the information.

4. A phlebotomist who attempts to collect a blood specimen (A) _____ the patient's

   (B) _____ can face a criminal charge of (C) _____ and (D) _____ as well as a

   (E) _____ suit for damages.

5. If a neglectful act occurs while an employee is doing something that is (A) _____ within his or her

   duties or (B) _____, the employee may be held (C) _____ (D) _____ for that act.

6. A hospital, as an (A) _____, cannot escape (B) _____ for a patient's injury simply by

   (C) _____ out various services to other persons and claiming it is not responsible because

   the party that caused the (D) _____ is not on its (E) _____.

7. If a phlebotomist tells a patient that he or she is going to collect a blood specimen, and the patient

   (A) _____ out an arm, it is considered (B) _____ (C) _____.

KNOWLEDGE DRILL 2-2: SCRAMBLED WORDS

Unscramble the following words using the hints given in parenthesis and the letters that have been placed in the correct boxes. Finish writing the correct spelling of the scrambled word in the corresponding boxes.

1. Aedtl _____ (this check helps ensure quality)

d				

2. Drisotacin _____ (used to monitor QA)

				c	a				

3. Fatpiflin _____ (an injured party)

	I			n				

4. Gingeencel _____ (not an issue if you are reasonable)

		g			g				

5. Hedlsorth _____ (exceeding this is not good)

	h			s				

6. Laquity _____ (must be assured in health care)

			I		t	

7. Savoriciu _____ (a kind of liability)

	i	c						

8. Talycodinfeitin _____ (privacy)

	o	n					i					

9. Ulastas _____ (a harmful touch)

	s	s				

10. Yencoptmec _____ (an educational standard)

		m		e		e			

KNOWLEDGE DRILL 2-3: TRUE/FALSE ACTIVITY

The following statements are all false. Circle the one or two words that make the statement false and write the correct word(s) that would make the statement true.

1. Documentation can be used for legal purposes as long as it is recent and includes only standard symbols.

2. A sentinel event (SE) is any unfavorable event that is unexpected and results in unremarkable or minor physical or psychological injury.

3. Use at least four ways to identify patients when providing laboratory services.

4. A CAP-certified laboratory also meets Medicare/Medicaid standards because CLIA grants reciprocity (mutual exchange of privileges) to CAP in the area of laboratory regulations.

5. CLSI's mission is *to develop clinical and laboratory programs and promote their curriculum worldwide.*

6. Quality indicators must be measurable, well defined, subjective, and nonspecific.

7. Instructions on how to prepare a patient for testing can be found by checking the laboratory's procedure manual.

8. The Joint Commission moved toward stricter patient ID requirements by their revision of CLSI standards in 2009.

9. Phlebotomist must "actively involve" nurses in their identification process during any specimen collection.

10. OSHA regulations require every business to have an infection control manual.

11. An IQCP form is to be completed when an occupational injury or exposure occurs.

12. Patient confidentiality is protected under federal law.

KNOWLEDGE DRILL 2-4: NATIONAL AGENCIES AND REGULATIONS

The following table identifies by name and abbreviation and summarizes the description, purpose, and functions of agencies and regulations described in Chapter 2 of the TEXTBOOK. Using the TEXTBOOK, fill in the blanks with the missing information.

Agency/Regulation Name/Abbreviation	Description	Purpose	Functions
1. The Joint (A) _____	An independent, (B) _____-_____-_____ organization	Establish (C) _____ for the operation of hospitals and other health-related facilities and services	• Key player in bringing (D) _____ _____ review techniques to health care • Oldest and largest (E) _____- _____ body in health care • Accredits and certifies more than (F) _____ health care organizations and programs in the United States
2. (A) _____ of American (B) _____	The membership in (C) _____ is (D) _____ board-certified (E) _____ and pathologists in training	Influence (F) _____ improvement in phlebotomy through (G) _____	• Offers (H) _____ _____ • Offers continuous form of laboratory (I) _____ by a team of pathologists and laboratory managers
3. (A) _____ and Laboratory (B) _____ Institute	A (C) _____, nonprofit, standards-developing organization with representatives from the (D) _____, industry, and government	Use a widespread agreement process to develop (E) _____ guidelines and standards for all areas of the laboratory	• Provides guidelines and standards on which phlebotomy program approval, (F) _____ examination questions, and the (G) _____ _____ _____ are based

4. (A) _____ Laboratory (B) _____ Amendments of 1988 | Federal regulations administered by the (C) _____ (abbreviation) whose regulations establish (D) _____ standards for all facilities that test (E) _____ specimens for the purpose of providing information used to diagnose, prevent, or treat disease or assess health status | To ensure the accuracy, (F) _____, and reliability of patient test results, regardless of the (G) _____, type, or size of the laboratory | • Provides (H) _____ and scientific (I) _____ and guidance
• Requires moderate and complex laboratory facilities to have routine inspections
• Requires (J) _____ protocols for all laboratory procedures

5. (A) _____ (B) _____ Agency for Clinical Laboratory Sciences | A recognized authority on quality (C) _____ laboratory education | Provides accreditation or (D) _____ for clinical laboratory education programs | • Provides external (E) _____ review of programs to determine if they meet certain established educational standards
• Requires that phlebotomy programs meet educational standards called (F) _____

KNOWLEDGE DRILL 2-5: CRIMINAL AND CIVIL ACTIONS

On the line provided, write the correct type of legal action (civil or criminal) associated with the descriptive statement.

1. _____ Punishable by fines and/or imprisonment

2. _____ Individual may be charged with a felony or a misdemeanor

3. _____ Involves injurious acts by others in society

4. _____ Concerned with actions between two private parties

5. _____ Monetary penalties awarded in a court of law

6. _____ Constitutes the bulk of legal actions dealt with health care

KNOWLEDGE DRILL 2-6: THE LITIGATION PROCESS

Number the following phases in the litigation process in chronological order from 1 through 7.

A. _____ A deposition is taken

B. _____ Appeal is filed by the losing party

C. _____ Attorney decides whether to take case or not

D. _____ Attorney files a complaint

E. _____ Injured party consults an attorney

F. _____ Patient becomes aware of prior possible injury

G. _____ Trial phase with judge and jury

KNOWLEDGE DRILL 2-7: GUIDELINES TO AVOID LAWSUITS

The following are statements concerning ways to avoid lawsuits. Finish each statement with the missing information from the TEXTBOOK.

1. Acquire informed consent _____

2. Be meticulous when _____

3. Carefully monitor the patient _____

4. Respect a patient's _____

5. Strictly adhere to CLSI standards _____

6. Use proper safety _____

7. Listen and respond appropriately to the _____

8. Accurately and legibly _____

9. Document _____

10. Participate in continuing education to _____

11. Perform at the prevailing _____

12. Never perform procedures that you are not _____

Skills Drills

SKILLS DRILL 2-1: REQUISITION ACTIVITY

Instructions: Answer the following questions concerning the test requisition shown below.

Any Hospital USA
1123 West Physician Drive
Any Town USA

Laboratory Test Requisition

- -

PATIENT INFORMATION:

Name: _____ Smith _____ John _____
             (last)   (first)   (MI)

Identification Number: __09365784__   Birth Date: __06/21/63__

Referring Physician: __Payne__

Date to be Collected: __03/15/15__   Time to be Collected: __0600__

Special Instructions: __line draw only__

- -

TEST(S) REQUIRED:

_____ NH4 – Ammonia	_____ Gluc – glucose
_____ Bili – Bilirubin, total & direct	_____ Hgb – hemoglobin
_____ BMP – basic metabolic panel	_____ Lact – lactic acid/lactate
_____ BUN – Blood urea nitrogen	_____ Plt. Ct. – platelet count
_____ Lytes – electrolytes	_____ PT – prothrombin time
_____ CBC – complete blood count	_____ PTT – partial thromboplastin time
_____ Chol – cholesterol	_____ RPR – rapid plasma regain
_____ ESR – erythrocyte sed rate	_____ T&S – type and screen
_____ EtOH – alcohol	_____ PSA – prostatic specific antigen
__X__ D-dimer	Other ___HIV_____

---

1. A new phlebotomist does not know anything about collecting a D-dimer or an HIV test. Where can the collection information on these tests be found?

2. What does patient consent involve when drawing an HIV sample?

SKILLS DRILL 2-2: WORD BUILDING

Divide each of the words below into all of its elements (parts): prefix (P), word root (WR), combining vowel (CV), and suffix (S). Write the word part and its definition on the corresponding lines. Write the general meaning of the word in the space provided. If the word does not have a particular element, write NA (not applicable) in its place.

Example: pathologists

Elements _____ / ____path____ / __o__ / _____logists_____
                          P   WR   CV   S

Definitions _____ / ____disease____ / _____ / ____specialist in the study of____

Meaning: a specialist who studies and interprets disease

1. Tachometer

   Elements _____ / _____ / _____ / _____
                            P   WR   CV   S

   Definitions _____ / _____ / _____ / _____

   Meaning:

2. Phlebotomy

   Elements _____ / _____ / _____ / _____
                            P   WR   CV   S

   Definitions _____ / _____ / _____ / _____

   Meaning:

3. Postanalytical

   Elements _____ / _____ / _____ / _____
                            P   WR   CV   S

   Definitions _____ / _____ / _____ / _____

   Meaning:

4. Chronology

   Elements _____ / _____ / _____ / _____
                            P   WR   CV   S

   Definitions _____ / _____ / _____ / _____

   Meaning:

SKILLS DRILL 2-3: CMS WEB SITE

Go to the Centers for Medicare & Medicaid Services Web site (CMS.gov). Click on the section "Outreach & Education." Under the heading REACH OUT, click on "Get digital media."

1. List the new medical resources now available for timely educational information.

   (1) _____

   (2) _____

   (3) _____

2. What do the Twitter accounts listed above offer?

   (1) _____

   _____

   (2) (a) _____

   (b) _____

SKILLS DRILL 2-4: QUEST DIAGNOSTICS WEB SITE

A. Go to the Quest Diagnostics-Official Site (questdiagnostic.com). Find the pull-down menu entitled **FOR PATIENTS.** Under the column **What We Offer,** choose **"Diagnostic Testing A-Z".** Scroll down to **TAKE ACTION** and click on **"Request a Test".**

   1. Can a person order their own blood work?

   2. How do they go about getting a desired test done?

   3. If your health care provider decides that the person should have this test, what is needed if a phlebotomist is not at that provider's site?

B. Under TOP QUESTIONS (upper left column), see "Does It Matter Which Lab I Choose?" List what Quest says are the six factors that are needed to be considered when choosing a laboratory.

   1. _____

   2. _____

   3. _____

   4. _____

   5. _____

   6. _____

Crossword

ACROSS

1. A type of negligence
3. Black stripes corresponding to letters and numbers
5. Person against whom the complaint is filed
9. Information collected for analysis
11. Clinical and Laboratory Sciences Institute
12. The state of being liable
13. Quality assurance (abbreviation)
14. Injured party in a lawsuit
17. Common name for complete test package
19. Where 10% of malpractice lawsuits end up
20. Complete medical file of a patient is called a _____
21. Level of normal care, _____ care
23. Anyone who has not reached age of majority
24. Begins legal proceedings
25. To give permission for medical procedure
26. Agency that manages federal HC programs (abbreviation)
27. A _____ of conduct
30. Type of legal action in which the party sues for monetary damages
33. National agency that accredits laboratory programs
35. _____ control or assurance
36. To examine and judge the worth of

DOWN

1. Provides health care to person over 65 years of age
2. Number of QA recommendations for CoWs
4. Federal rules and regulations for all diagnostic laboratories
6. Check that compares current results with previous ones
7. Turnaround time
8 A process used to settle disputes
10. Follow a path by means of evidence to get to outcome
14. Lawyers are said to _____ law
15. Realities or truths
16. To do damage or injury
18. General course or drift (pl)
21. Taking deposition and interrogating persons
22. Another abbreviation for SGOT
27. Hematoma/injury and discoloring of skin
28. Intentional threat of immediate harm
29. Deceitful practice
31. Based on the law
32. Use of checks and controls (abbreviation)
34. Chance of injury, damage, or loss

Chapter Review Questions

1. This organization establishes standards for the operation of hospitals and other health care facilities and services.
   a. American Hospital Association
   b. College of American Pathology
   c. National Accrediting Agency
   d. The Joint Commission

2. An agency that manages the federal health care programs of Medicare and Medicaid is the:
   a. CAP.
   b. CLIA.
   c. CLSI.
   d. CMS.

3. This is an early warning policy to help health care organizations identify unfavorable actions and take steps to prevent them.
   a. Quality indicators
   b. Sentinel events
   c. Six Sigma
   d. Threshold values

4. These measurable, objective guides are established to monitor all aspects of patient care.
   a. Indicators
   b. Outcomes
   c. Policies
   d. Procedures

5. Which manual describes the chemical, electrical, and radiation concerns for the laboratory?
   a. Infection control manual
   b. Procedure manual
   c. Safety manual
   d. Test catalog

6. One of the generic steps in risk management is
   a. assessment of test menus.
   b. education of the employees.
   c. evaluation of medical records.
   d. review of employees' records.

7. Informed consent means that:
   a. a patient's medical records are available for review by all health care workers.
   b. all consequences of a medical procedure have been given to the patient.
   c. the patient received a book outlining all procedures and their consequences.
   d. the patient's confidentiality has been breached during the assessment process.

8. This national organization develops guidelines and sets standards for laboratory procedures.
   a. CAP
   b. CLIAC
   c. CLSI
   d. NAACLS

9. A phlebotomist hired by a hospital as a temporary employee commits a negligent act for which the hospital is liable. This is an example of:
   a. assault and battery.
   b. *res ipsa loquitur.*
   c. *respondeat superior.*
   d. standard of care.

10. A phlebotomist collects a sample from a 16-year-old patient without obtaining parental or guardian consent. The phlebotomist could be charged with which of the following?
    a. Assault and battery
    b. Invasion of privacy
    c. Statute of limitations
    d. Vicarious liability

11. National Patient Safety Goals (NPSGs) are:
    a. rules set down by CDC and overseen by OSHA.
    b. standards set by NAACLS for educational programs.
    c. the Joint Commission's specific safety requirements.
    d. voluntary guidelines and protocol written by CLSI.

12. A comparison of current test results with previous results for the same test on the same patient is called a
    a. delta check.
    b. quality indicator.
    c. risk control.
    d. sentinel event.

13. Which one of the following forms states the concern and describes the corrective action when a problem occurs?
    a. Equipment check form
    b. Delta review form
    c. Internal report
    d. Quality control check

14. A type of negligence committed by a professional is called
    a. assault.
    b. battery.
    c. invasion of privacy.
    d. malpractice.

15. Failure to keep privileged medical information private is
    a. breach of confidentiality.
    b. invasion of privacy.
    c. *res ipsa loquitur.*
    d. vicarious liability.

16. Risk factors in phlebotomy can be identified by
    a. adhering to national standards of good practice.
    b. consistently following OSHA guidelines.
    c. looking at trends in internal reporting forms.
    d. managing patient safety and sentinel events.

17. One of TJC's 2014 safety goals for the clinical laboratory states:
    a. standardize all outpatient phlebotomy practices.
    b. improve the turn around time for test results.
    c. sanitize collection carts and equipment daily.
    d. label all specimens before leaving the patient.

18. EMR stands for
    a. electronic Medical Record.
    b. emergency Medical Radiofrequency.
    c. employee Medical Restrictions.
    d. equipment Manufacturer's Rating.

19. A phlebotomist using an armband for patient ID must also
    a. check the room number for additional verification.
    b. have the patient state additional ID information.
    c. make certain requisition matches wristband.
    d. write down location of the patient on the requisition.

20. Within the ACOs, there is a requirement to
    a. decrease patient visits due to federal oversite.
    b. duplicate patient information for other physicians.
    c. increase patient load in each physician's offices.
    d. share patients' information with all participants.

Case Studies

Case Study 2-1: Quality Assurance in a CoW Laboratory

The CoW laboratory in a large internal medicine group practice performed over 50 waived tests a day. The medical assistants and the phlebotomists who performed the waived testing were all trained OJTs. It was obvious from the inconsistent results recorded on the cumulative report that everyone's technique differed somewhat. When notification came from CLIA that they would be visiting the site within the next month, the lead physician decided that a QA process had to be put into place. He directed the laboratory staff to the CLIA Web site for instructions on waived testing standardization in the form of GLPs issued by CLIAC.

QUESTIONS

1. What are CLIA and CLIAC?

2. Why is CLIA visiting their site?

3. What are the GLPs and what makes them valuable in standardizing the waived testing process?

4. What are other examples of QC components that could be put in place in this laboratory setting?

Case Study 2-2: Blood Draw Fails Delta Check

It was a very busy day in the hospital laboratory since two phlebotomists were out for medical reasons. An order came from the fourth floor for a timed draw. Joe, a phlebotomist from a temporary agency, was still there, even though he was supposed to have gotten off 2 hours earlier. No one was there to collect the specimen except Joe. Knowing how important it was, he decided to go ahead and collect it. When he arrived in the room, the patient was seated in a chair between the beds. Joe asked the patient his name and in which bed he belonged. When the seated patient answered with the right last name and pointed to the correct bed, Joe proceeded to collect the specimen from him while he sat in the chair. Joe labeled the specimen tubes at the nursing station while noting the draw on the desk clipboard. When a second specimen was drawn from

the patient later that morning, it failed the delta check. The second specimen was recollected and the results showed the specimen that Joe had drawn to be in error.

QUESTIONS

1. What is a delta check?

2. What do you see that could have caused this discrepancy?

3. What should Joe have done differently?

4. What were Joe's obligations to the laboratory after his regular shift?

5. Who is ultimately responsible for Joe's actions while he is at work?

Case Study 2-3: Nerve Injury

A phlebotomist prepares to draw three tubes of blood from an outpatient. The only vein that is visible is the basilic vein on the right arm. He was taught that the basilic vein is the last choice for venipuncture because it is hard to anchor and a major nerve lies close to it, but it is so large he decides that he can draw it without a problem. When he inserts the needle, sure enough, the vein rolls and the needle slips beside the vein. The patient cries out in pain, and jerks her arm. The needle goes even deeper, but blood begins to flow into the tube, so he continues the draw. The patient tells him it is hurting and to pull the needle out, but the tubes are filling quickly, so he continues to fill all three before ending the draw. The woman is still in pain and her arm begins to swell

in the area of the draw. The phlebotomist quickly wraps a pressure bandage around the arm and tells her she is free to go. The patient is later diagnosed with permanent nerve injury and sues the clinic.

QUESTIONS

1. Can the phlebotomist be held liable for the woman's injury?

2. What tort might be involved in this case?

3. Do you think the standard of care was breached? Why or why not?

Chapter 3

Infection Control, Safety, First Aid, and Personal Wellness

Objectives

Study the information in the TEXTBOOK that corresponds to each objective to prepare yourself for the activities in this chapter.

1 Demonstrate knowledge of terminology and practices related to Infection Control and identify agencies associated with infection control precautions, procedures and programs.

2 Identify key elements of the Bloodborne Pathogen Standard and the Needlestick Safety and Prevention Act, and identify associated organizations.

3 Identify hazards, warning symbols, and safety rules related to the laboratory, patient areas, and biological, electrical, fire, radiation, and chemical safety, and discuss actions to take if incidents occur.

4 Recognize symptoms needing first aid and list the main points of the American Heart Association CPR and ECC guidelines.

5 Describe the role of personal wellness as it relates to nutrition, rest, exercise, stress management and back protection.

Matching

Use choices only once unless otherwise indicated.

MATCHING 3-1: KEY TERMS AND DESCRIPTIONS

Match each key term with the *best* description.

Key Terms (1–20)

1. _____ Asepsis
2. _____ BBP
3. _____ Biohazard
4. _____ CDC
5. _____ Chain of infection
6. _____ Engineering controls
7. _____ EPA
8. _____ Fire tetrahedron
9. _____ Fomites
10. _____ HAI
11. _____ HBV
12. _____ HCS
13. _____ HCV
14. _____ HICPAC
15. _____ HIV
16. _____ Immune
17. _____ Infectious/causative agent
18. _____ Isolation procedures
19. _____ Microbe
20. _____ Neutropenic

Descriptions

A. A series of events that lead to infection
B. Anything harmful to health
C. Chemistry of fire representation
D. Condition of being free of pathogenic microbes
E. Devices that isolate a workplace BBP hazard
F. Federal agency charged with the investigation and control of various diseases
G. Federal agency that regulates the disposal of hazardous waste
H. Federal organization that advises the CDC on nosocomial infection–prevention guidelines
I. Having an abnormally low neutrophil count
J. Hepatitis B virus
K. Hepatitis C virus
L. Inanimate objects that can harbor material containing infectious agents
M. Infection acquired in any health care setting
N. OSHA standard regarding hazardous chemicals
O. Pathogen responsible for causing an infection
P. Procedures that separate patients with certain transmissible infections from others
Q. Protected from a particular disease by antibodies
R. Short for microorganism
S. Term applied to infectious microorganisms in blood and other body fluids
T. Virus that causes AIDS

Key Terms (21–40)

21. _____ NHSN
22. _____ NIOSH
23. _____ Nosocomial infection
24. _____ OSHA
25. _____ Parenteral
26. _____ Pathogenic
27. _____ Pathogens
28. _____ Percutaneous
29. _____ Permucosal

Descriptions

A. Any route other than the digestive tract
B. Capable of causing disease
C. Contains hazardous chemical information
D. Federal agency that recommends ways to prevent work-related injury
E. Federal agency that mandates and enforces safe working conditions for employees
F. Individual with little resistance to an infectious agent
G. Infection acquired in a hospital
H. Microorganisms capable of causing disease
I. Practices that reduce the likelihood of BBP exposure
J. Precautions that reduce the risk of airborne, droplet, or contact transmission

30. _____ Pictogram

31. _____ PPE

32. _____ Reservoir

33. _____ Reverse isolation

34. _____ SDS

35. _____ Standard precautions

36. _____ Susceptible host

37. _____ Transmission-based precautions

38. _____ Vector transmission

39. _____ Vehicle transmission

40. _____ Work practice controls

K. Precautions to be used in caring for all patients

L. Protective items worn by an individual

M. Protects a patient who is highly susceptible to infection

N. Provides a widely used HAI tracking System

O. Source of an infectious microorganism

P. Through mucous membranes

Q. Through the skin

R. Transmission of an infectious agent by an insect, arthropod, or animal

S. Transmission of an infectious agent through contaminated food, water, drugs, or blood

T. Universally accepted hazard symbol

MATCHING 3-2: ACTIVITY EXAMPLE AND MEANS OF TRANSMISSION

Draw an arrow from the example of an activity that could lead to infection in the first column to the most likely means of transmission that would be involved in the second column. Use a different colored pen or pencil for each arrow. Answers can be used only once.

Activity Example

1. Collecting a throat culture specimen from a coughing patient without wearing a mask

2. Entering a TB patient's room without an N95 respirator

3. Filling a TB test syringe with antigen without first cleaning the top of the antigen vial

4. Handling a dead rodent

5. Kissing someone with mononucleosis

6. Rubbing your eye after touching a contaminated blood tube

Means of Transmission

A. Airborne

B. Direct contact

C. Indirect contact

D. Droplet

E. Vector

F. Vehicle

MATCHING 3-3: CLASS OF FIRE, TYPE OF MATERIAL, AND METHOD REQUIRED TO EXTINGUISH

Using a different colored pen or pencil for each class of fire, draw an arrow from the class of fire in the first column to the type of materials involved in the second column. Using the same color used for the class of fire, draw an arrow from the type of material involved to the method required to extinguish the fire found in the third column.

Class of Fire	Type of Material	Method Required to Extinguish
Class A	1. Combustible metals	A. Block oxygen source or smother
Class B	2. Electrical equipment	B. Cool and smother with splash prevention agent
Class C	3. Flammable liquid	C. Cool with water or water-based solution
Class D	4. Cooking oils	D. Extinguish with dry powder agent or sand
Class K	5. Wood or paper	E. Extinguish with nonconducting agent

MATCHING 3-4: TYPE OF SPILL AND CLEANUP PROCEDURE

Match the type of spill with the cleanup procedure (Procedure 3–2).

Type of Spill

1. _____ Small spill (a few drops)

2. _____ Large spill

3. _____ Dried spill

4. _____ Spill involving broken glass

Cleanup Procedure

A. Carefully absorb spill with a paper towel or similar material. Discard material in a biohazard waste container. Clean area with appropriate disinfectant.

B. Moisten spill with disinfectant (avoid scraping, which could disperse infectious organisms into the air). Absorb spill with paper towel or similar material. Discard material in a biohazard waste container. Clean area with appropriate disinfectant.

C. Use a special clay or chlorine-based powder to absorb or gel (thicken) the liquid. Scoop or sweep up absorbed or thickened material. Discard material in a biohazard waste container. Wipe spill area with appropriate disinfectant.

D. Wear heavy-duty utility gloves. Scoop or sweep up material. Discard in a biohazard sharps container. Clean area with appropriate disinfectant.

MATCHING 3-5: HCN PICTOGRAMS

The following are nine GHS hazard category pictograms. Match the pictogram to the example of the type of hazard it represents. Put an X in parenthesis next to the one pictogram that is not an HCS pictogram.

Pictogram

1. _____

2. _____

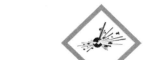

3. _____

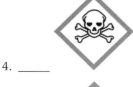

4. _____

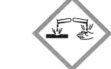

5. _____

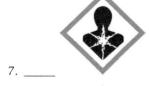

6. _____

7. _____

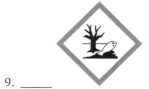

8. _____

9. _____

Hazard Example

A. Acute toxicity (fatal or toxic)

B. Aquatic toxicity

C. Carcinogen

D. Explosives

E. Eye damage

F. Flammables

G. Gases under pressure

H. Oxidizers

I. Respiratory tract irritant

Labeling Exercises

LABELING EXERCISE 3-1: NFPA 704 MARKING SYSTEM

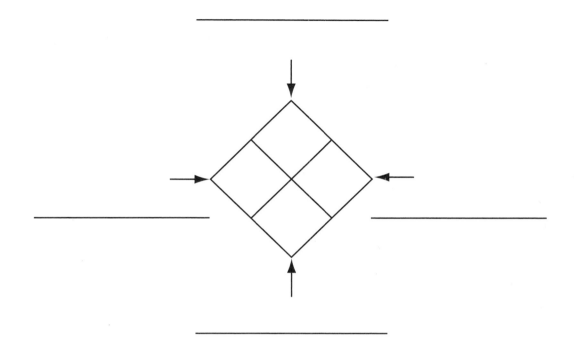

Label the quadrants in the NFPA marking system diagram above according to the type of hazard they identify. Color the quadrants the appropriate color code (one quadrant will remain uncolored). Using a black marker, write the signal number (or draw the symbol if applicable) for each of the following hazards in the appropriate quadrant:

- Material that on short exposure could cause serious temporary injury even with prompt medical attention

- Material that would have to be preheated before ignition could occur

- Material that is capable of detonating or exploding at normal temperature and pressure

- Material that is radioactive

LABELING EXERCISE 3-2: ENGINEERING CONTROLS AND WORK PRACTICE CONTROLS

Each illustration below shows an item (or items) or a practice that is either an engineering control, work practice control, or both. Write the name of the item(s) or practice shown followed by the type of control it is, on the corresponding line beneath the illustration.

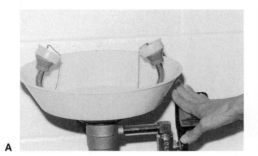 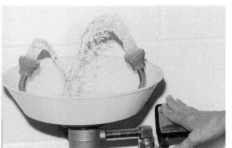

1. _____

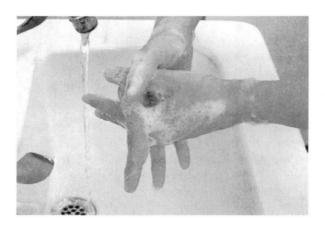

2. _____

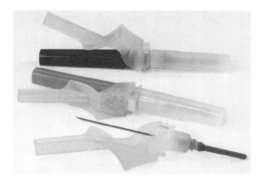

3. _____

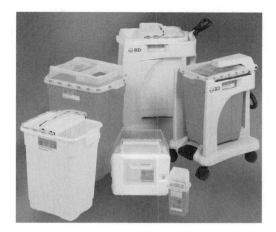

4. _____

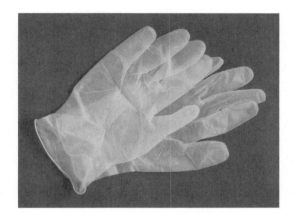

5. _____

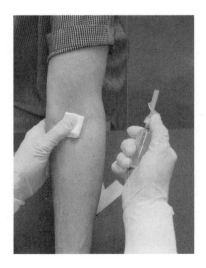

6. _____

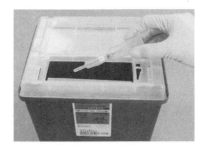

7. _____

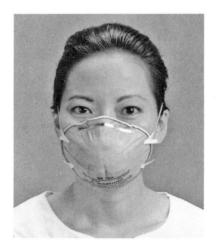

8. _____

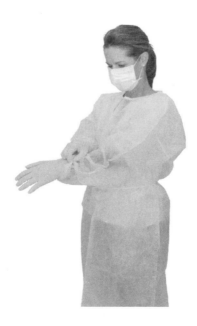

9. _____

Knowledge Drills

KNOWLEDGE DRILL 3-1: CAUTION AND KEY POINT RECOGNITION

The following sentences are taken from selected "CAUTION and KEY POINT" statements found throughout Chapter 3 in the TEXTBOOK. Using the TEXTBOOK, fill in the blanks with the missing information.

1. The transmission of (A) _____ viruses and (B) _____ through blood transfusion is also considered (C) _____ transmission.

2. (A) _____ transmission differs from airborne transmission in that (B) _____ normally travel less than (C) _____ and do not remain (D) _____ in the air.

3. Individuals who are exposed to the (A) _____ _____ (_____) are less likely to contract the disease if they have previously completed an (B) _____ (C) _____ series.

4. (A) _____ regulations require employers to offer (B) _____ (C) _____ free of charge to employees whose duties involve risk of (D) _____.

5. The (A) _____ _____ _____ (___) consensus recommendations in the 2009 *Guidelines on Hand Hygiene in Health Care* are that (B) _____ do not wear artificial (C) _____ (D) _____ when having direct contact with patients, and natural nails should be kept short (0.5 cm long or approximately (E) _____ long).

6. Wearing (A) _____ during phlebotomy procedures is (B) _____ by the OSHA (C) _____ _____ _____.

7. The (A) _____ is known as "the right to know law" because the (B) _____ requirement gives employees the right to know about the (C) _____ (D) _____ they encounter in the workplace.

8. The original compress should not be removed when adding (A) _____ ones because removal can (B) _____ the (C) _____ process.

9. *Never* give fluids if the patient is (A) _____ or (B) _____ or has injuries likely to require (C) _____ and anesthesia.

10. According to the American Heart Association, if activity during work is low to moderate a 30-minute (A) _____ _____ or similar exercise (B) _____ can improve blood pressure and reduce the risk of (C) _____ _____ and (D) _____ _____.

11. In addition, if hands are heavily contaminated with (A) _____ material and hand washing facilities are not available, it is recommended that hands be cleaned with (B) _____ - _____ _____ followed by the use of an (C) _____ - _____ antiseptic hand cleaner.

12. The most common type of (A) _____ reported to NHSN is (B) _____ _____ _____ (___), accounting for over (C) _____ of all HAIs.

KNOWLEDGE DRILL 3-2: SCRAMBLED WORDS

Use each numbered hint below to unscramble the words listed after it. Write the correct spelling of the scrambled word on the line next to it.

1. Three types of biohazard exposure routes

   a. merpuscola

		r		u		o			

   b. troucanesupe

	e				t			e		u	

   c. tegionnis

	n	g			t	i		

2. Together they create the need for a fire extinguisher

   a. teha

		a	

   b. genoxy

		y		e	

   c. lufe

	u		

   d. mechlica noriteac

		e		i		a	

	e		c	t			

3. They play a role in radiation exposure

   a. miet

			e

   b. gleindish

		i			d			g

   c. staindec

	i		t				e

4. A chemical safety requirement

   a. yesfat

	a			t	

   b. taad

	a		

   c. hetse

		e		t

5. A symptom of shock (three word phrase)

a. pardi

			i	

b. akew

			k

c. slupe

				e

6. They play a role in personal wellness

a. sciereex

		e			i		e	

b. tunionirt

			r	i		i		

c. neighey

		g			n	

KNOWLEDGE DRILL 3-3: BREAKING THE CHAIN OF INFECTION (Box 3-1)

List five things a phlebotomist can personally do to break the chain of infection.

1. _____

2. _____

3. _____

4. _____

5. _____

KNOWLEDGE DRILL 3-4: SITUATIONS THAT REQUIRE HAND HYGIENE

The following are statements concerning situations that require hand washing. Fill in the blanks with the missing information.

1. Before and after each _____

2. Between _____ procedures on a patient such as wound care and drawing blood

3. Before putting on gloves and _____

4. Before leaving the _____

5. Before going to lunch or on _____

6. Before and after going to the _____

7. Whenever hands become _____ contaminated

KNOWLEDGE DRILL 3-5: SAFETY RULES WHEN IN PATIENT ROOMS AND OTHER PATIENT AREAS

The following are safety rules to follow when in patient rooms and other patient areas. After each rule, list at least one reason why it should be followed.

1. Avoid running. _____

_____

2. Be careful entering and exiting patient rooms. _____

3. Do not touch electrical equipment in patient rooms while drawing blood. _____

_____

4. Follow standard precautions when handling specimens. _____

_____

5. Replace bed rails that were let down during patient procedures. _____

KNOWLEDGE DRILL 3-6: PATHOGEN TRANSMISSION AND PRECAUTIONS

A list of microorganisms, diseases, and conditions follows. Using colored pens or pencils write the type of precautions involved. Write "A" in blue if airborne precautions are required, "C" in black if contact precautions are required, "D" in green if droplet precautions are required, and "S" in brown next to those that require only standard precautions. Write BBP in red next to those that are also bloodborne pathogens.

1. _____ *Bordetella pertussis*

2. _____ *C. difficile*

3. _____ CMV

4. _____ Group A strep (draining wound)

5. _____ HBV

6. _____ HCV

7. _____ HIV

8. _____ HDV

9. _____ Impetigo

10. _____ Influenza

11. _____ Malaria-causing microbe

12. _____ *Mycoplasma pneumoniae*

13. _____ *Neisseria meningitides*

14. _____ RSV

15. _____ Rubella virus (congenital)

16. _____ Rubeola virus

17. _____ *Staphylococcus aureus* (draining abscess)

18. _____ Syphilis-causing microbe

19. _____ *Mycobacterium tuberculosis*

20. _____ Varicella virus

KNOWLEDGE DRILL 3-7: TRUE/FALSE ACTIVITY

The following statements are all false. Circle the one or two word(s) that make the statement false and write the correct word(s) that would make the statement true, in the space provided.

1. Asepsis is a condition of being contaminated with microorganisms that can cause disease.

2. Nosocomial infection is a relatively new term applied to infections acquired during health care delivery in any health care setting.

3. The HCS was developed to protect employees from bloodborne pathogens.

4. The source of an infectious agent is called a vector.

5. OSHA regulations require employers to offer reduced price HBV vaccination for employees whose duties involve risk of exposure.

6. Studies have shown that artificial nails harbor fewer pathogenic microbes than natural nails.

7. The spores of *Clostridium difficile* are easily killed by alcohol-based hand cleaners.

8. According to CLSI guidelines, pants worn by laboratory personnel should be ½ to 1½ inches off the floor to prevent contamination.

9. Except for a mask, PPE worn in isolation rooms is removed at the door before leaving.

10. Transmission-based precautions are to be used in the care of all patients.

11. A signal word specifies the reactivity of a hazard.

12. Pictograms are round with a red border.

Skills Drills

SKILLS DRILL 3-1: REQUISITION ACTIVITY

Any Hospital USA
1123 West Physician Drive
Any Town USA

Laboratory Test Requisition

- -

PATIENT INFORMATION:

Name: _____ Doe _____ Jane _____
                (last)   (first)   (MI)
Identification Number: __093656321_____ Birth Date: _04/11/68_____

Referring Physician: __Payne_____

Date to be Collected: __03/15/15_____ Time to be Collected: ___0600_____

Special Instructions: _____

- -

TEST(S) REQUIRED:

_____ NH4 – Ammonia	_____ Gluc – glucose
_____ Bili – Bilirubin, total & direct	_____ Hgb – hemoglobin
_____ BMP – basic metabolic panel	_____ Lact – lactic acid/lactate
_____ BUN – Blood urea nitrogen	_____ Plt. Ct. – platelet count
_____ Lytes – electrolytes	_____ PT – prothrombin time
__X__ CBC – complete blood count	_____ PTT – partial thromboplastin time
_____ Chol – cholesterol	_____ RPR – rapid plasma reagin
__X__ ESR – erythrocyte sed rate	_____ T&S – type and screen
_____ ETOH – alcohol	_____ PSA – prostatic specific antigen
_____ D-dimer	Other __AFB culture_____

A phlebotomist is sent to collect the specimens on the following requisition. Upon arrival at the patient's room, he finds an airborne precautions sign on the door.

1. What precautions, if any, must the phlebotomist take before entering the room?

2. Which test requested might be a clue as to why the patient has airborne precautions?

3. What is the full name of the correct answer to 2 and why is it a clue to required precautions?

4. Name the disease the patient has, or is suspected of having?

SKILLS DRILL 3-2: WORD BUILDING

Divide each word below into all of its elements (parts): prefix (P), word root (WR), combining vowel (CV), and suffix (S). Write the word part and its definition on the corresponding lines. Write the general meaning of the word in the space provided. If the word does not have a particular element, write NA (not applicable) in its place.

Example: Neonatal

Elements _____*neo*_____ / _____*nat*_____ / _____ / _____*al*_____
                        P   WR   CV   S

Definitions _____*new*_____ / _____*birth*_____ / _____ / _____*pertaining to*_____

Meaning: pertaining to a newborn

1. Asepsis

   Elements _____ / _____ / _____ / _____
                 P   WR   CV   S

   Definition _____ / _____ / _____ / _____ / _____

   Meaning:

2. Cardiopulmonary

   Elements _____ / _____ / _____ / _____ / _____
                 P   WR   CV   WR   S

   Definition _____ / _____ / _____ / _____ / _____

   Meaning:

3. Dermatitis

   Elements _____ / _____ / _____ / _____ / _____
                 P   WR   CV   S

   Definition _____ / _____ / _____ / _____ / _____

   Meaning:

4. Hemorrhage

   Elements _____ / _____ / _____ / _____ / _____
                 P   WR   CV   S

   Definition _____ / _____ / _____ / _____ / _____

   Meaning:

5. Hepatitis

   Elements _____ / _____ / _____ / _____ / _____
                 P   WR   CV   S

   Definition _____ / _____ / _____ / _____ / _____

   Meaning:

6. Percutaneous

   Elements _____ / _____ / _____ / _____ / _____
                 P   WR   CV   S

   Definition _____ / _____ / _____ / _____ / _____

   Meaning:

SKILLS DRILL 3-3: HAND WASHING TECHNIQUE (Procedure 3-1)

Fill in the blanks with the missing information.

Step	**Explanation/Rationale**
1. Stand back so that you do not (A) _____ _____ _____.	The (B) _____ may be (C) _____.
2. Turn on the faucet and (D) _____ _____ under warm, running water.	Water should not be too hot or (E) _____ _____ and hands should be (F) _____ before applying (G) _____ to minimize drying, chapping, or cracking of hands from frequent hand washing.
3. Apply soap and work up a (H) _____.	A good (I) _____ is needed to reach all surfaces.
4. Scrub all surfaces, including between the fingers and around the (J) _____.	Scrubbing is necessary to dislodge (K) _____ from surfaces, especially between fingers and around (L) _____.
5. Rub your hands together (M) _____.	Friction helps loosen dead skin, dirt, debris, and (N) _____. (Steps 4 and 5 should take at least (O) _____, about the time it takes to sing the (P) _____.)
6. Rinse your hands in a (Q) _____ motion from (R) _____ to (S) _____.	Rinsing with the hands (T) _____ allows (U) _____ to be (V) _____ _____ the hands and fingers into the sink rather than flowing (W) _____ _____ the arm or wrist.
7. Dry hands with a (X) _____ paper towel.	Hands must be dried thoroughly and gently to prevent chapping or cracking. (Y) _____ towels can be a source of (Z)_____.
8. Use a (AA) _____ paper towel to (BB) _____ _____ _____ _____ unless it is foot or motion activated.	Clean hands should not touch contaminated (CC)_____ _____.

Crossword

ACROSS

1. Condition showing decreased amount of neutrophils
5. Type of fire, _____ A, B, C, D, or K
8. Bio_____, cautious handling of biological materials
9. Type of isolation system
10. Capable of living
11. Pathway link in the chain of infection
12. Federal agency charged with controlling disease
13. Infectious insect, arthropod, or animal
15. Tuberculosis
16. Tuberculin test
18. PPE facial covering
19. Results from insufficient blood flow to the heart
20. Most frequently occurring laboratory-related blood-borne pathogen
21. Infection acquired in the hospital
23. Resistant to a disease
26. Code used to remember how to operate a fire extinguisher
27. Injection to prevent acquiring a disease
28. AIDS virus
29. Institute requiring N95 respirator for HCWs who may encounter airborne contaminants
31. Precautions to follow for all patients
34. Intravenous (abbrev.)
35. Strategy to prevent exposure to BBPs (abbrev.)
37. Environmental protection agency (abbrev.)
38. Institute that suggests a predominantly plant-based diet
39. Protective covering for skin and clothing
40. Percutaneous means through the_____

DOWN

2. Work practice and _____ controls
3. An N95 respirator must be worn around a patient with this disease
4. Cause to become diseased with virus or bacteria
5. _____ of infection
6. Having little resistance to infection or disease
7. Basin for flushing eye after contamination
14. Process of passing disease from one to another
17. Unit in a hospital where intensive care is given
18. Microscopic organism
22. An example of PPE clothing worn over scrubs
24. Most common type of HAI
25. PPEs for hands
26. Items worn to protect an individual from infectious substances
27. Type of agent for hepatitis disease
28. Anyone infected with HBV is at risk for acquiring this virus
29. Agency that regulates fire codes
30. Most widespread chronic BBP illness in the United States
32. Term for a microbe that causes an infection
33. Chance of injury, damage or loss
36. Federal agency dealing with transportation

Chapter Review Questions

1. Terms used to identify components of the chain of infection include
   a. Infectious agent
   b. Susceptible host
   c. Reservoir
   d. All of the above

2. Which of the following is an example of employee screening for infection control?
   a. HBV vaccination
   b. MMR vaccination
   c. TB testing
   d. All of the above

3. CDC and HICPAC recommendations allow the use of alcohol-based antiseptic hand cleaners in place of hand washing as long as
   a. gloves were worn during the prior activity.
   b. hands are first cleaned with detergent wipes.
   c. hands have no visible dirt or organic material.
   d. all of the above conditions are met.

4. Standard precautions
   a. apply only to secretions and excretions that contain blood.
   b. are to be used when caring for all patients at all times.
   c. never supersede other CDC isolation recommendations.
   d. should not be combined with other precautions.

5. Which of the following actions would violate a laboratory safety rule?
   a. Chewing gum while processing specimens
   b. Keeping food in a laboratory reagent refrigerator
   c. Wearing artificial nails
   d. All of the above

6. Which of the following is an example of a blood-borne pathogen?
   a. Cytomegalovirus
   b. Group A strep
   c. TB mycobacterium
   d. Varicella virus

7. Which of the following meet the OSHA BBP standard definition of an engineering control?
   a. Self-sheathing needle
   b. Sharps container
   c. Splash shield
   d. All of the above

8. The best defense against HBV infection is:
   a. HBV vaccination.
   b. proper hand hygiene.
   c. using safety needles.
   d. wearing gloves.

9. Which of the following involves the possibility of a permucosal BBP exposure?
   a. Failing to cover broken skin with a bandage
   b. Getting stuck with a used phlebotomy needle
   c. Licking the fingers to turn laboratory manual pages
   d. Opening blood tubes without a safety shield

10. Proper procedure for cleaning the site of an injury from a contaminated needle includes
    a. cleaning it with povidone–iodine or another antiseptic.
    b. squeezing the injured area hard until it bleeds freely.
    c. washing it with soap and water for at least 30 seconds.
    d. all of the above.

11. Class "C" fires occur with
    a. ordinary combustibles.
    b. flammable liquids.
    c. electrical equipment.
    d. reactive metals.

12. Normally the most effective means of controlling external hemorrhage is
    a. application of a tourniquet.
    b. applying firm direct pressure.
    c. finger pressure over an artery.
    d. holding an ice pack on the site.

13. In the event of a chemical splash to the eyes, they should be flushed with water for a minimum of
    a. 2 minutes.
    b. 5 minutes.
    c. 10 minutes.
    d. 15 minutes.

14. In the NFPA 704 marking system, health hazards are indicated in the
    a. blue quadrant on the left.
    b. red quadrant at the top.
    c. yellow quadrant on the right.
    d. white quadrant on the bottom.

15. Approximately 20% of all workplace injuries involve
    a. back injuries.
    b. foot problems.
    c. needlesticks.
    d. stress reactions.

16. The most common type of HAI reported to NHSN is
    a. central line infection.
    b. respiratory infection.
    c. surgical site infection.
    d. urinary tract infection.

17. A phlebotomist whose hands are visibly contaminated should:
    a. clean them using alcohol wipes.
    b. scrub them with hand cleaner.
    c. wash them with soap and water.
    d. wipe them with detergent wipes.

18. One of the newest challenges in antibiotic resistance is
    a. *Clostridium difficile*
    b. group A streptococcus
    c. methicillin-resistant *Staphylococcus aureus*
    d. multidrug-resistant gram-negative bacteria

19. The pictogram for this type of hazard is an exclamation point.
    a. corrosion   c. flammable
    b. eye irritant   d. pyrophoric

20. Holistic comes from the Greek word *Holos,* which means to
    a. heal.   c. nourish.
    b. mend.   d. restore.

Case Studies

Case Study 3-1: Airborne Precautions

A phlebotomist arrives at a patient's room for a timed blood draw. She observes an airborne precautions sign on the patient's door. There is a cart in the hallway outside the door with supplies on it.

QUESTIONS

1. What will the phlebotomist have to do before she enters the room?

2. Will the specimen require special handling in addition to what is normally required for the test?

3. Name one disease that requires airborne precautions for anyone entering the patient's room.

4. Name two diseases that do not require airborne precautions for a phlebotomist who is immune to them.

Case Study 3-2: Work Restrictions (Appendix D)

A phlebotomist wakes up with a fever and an extremely sore throat. He calls his physician who sends him to a laboratory for a rapid strep test. The test is positive for group A strep. The physician gives him a prescription for an antibiotic. The phlebotomist picks up the prescription and takes the first dose at 13:00 hours. He is scheduled to work later that afternoon. He has used all his sick leave, so he takes some aspirin and goes to work.

QUESTIONS

1. What work restrictions are required for a person with strep throat?

2. What is the earliest that he should have reported for work provided he was symptom free?

3. What might be the consequences of reporting to work when he still had symptoms?

Case Study 3-3: Traveling Germs

A phlebotomist works the morning shift at a large hospital. Today he is wearing a brand new pair of scrubs his wife just bought for him the day before. They are a little long, so he rolls them up. Unfortunately they do not stay that way and he finally just lets them drag the floor. He considers his scrubs street clothes since he always remembers to wear his lab coat when drawing patients. Several of his patients have been in contact isolation today. He has been careful to follow all precautions indicated. Two rooms have a sign on the door that says hand washing with soap and water is required after patient contact, and he has done so meticulously. When his shift is over he stops by the daycare center to pick up his 3-year old son. While there he talks with a neighbor who is there to pick up her toddler. The toddler is sucking on a pacifier while holding onto his mother's legs, begging to be picked up. The pacifier drops on the floor next to the phlebotomist's feet. Before his mom has a chance to retrieve it, the toddler picks it up and puts it in his mouth.

The next week he learns that the neighbor's toddler has been hospitalized due to severe diarrhea and dehydration.

QUESTIONS

1. Why would hand washing with soap and water be required in addition to the contact precautions required for several of the patients?

2. What CLSI guideline was not been followed by the phlebotomist?

3. The phlebotomist could have had something to do with the toddler's illness. Why is that?

4. If the phlebotomist was responsible for the toddler's illness, what can he do to prevent something similar from happening in the future?

Case Study 3-4: Trash Bin Fire

Just as a phlebotomist arrives at work and comes through the door, the fire alarm sounds, the fire sprinkler system in the hallway activates, and the door down the hall automatically shuts. There is a trash bin near the door with heavy smoke and flames coming from it. Since it is partially covered, the water has little effect on the fire. No one else is in sight. The phlebotomist runs to a fire extinguisher nearby, grabs it, pulls the pin, and puts the fire out. It does not appear to have spread beyond the trash bin. Just then the firemen arrive on the scene.

QUESTIONS

1. What class of fire was most likely involved in this incident and why?

2. What type of extinguisher would be required to put it out?

3. The fire extinguisher in the hall was most likely what type?

4. What may have caused the fire?

5. What is the code word for action in the event of a fire and what does it mean?

Unit I Crossword Exercise

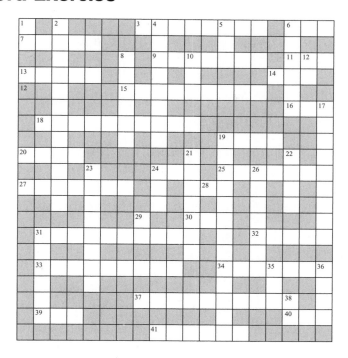

ACROSS

3. Disease transmission by aerosols of infectious agents that are inhaled
6. Infection acquired in any health care setting
7. *Exsanguinated* means that all of this is removed
9. Inanimate objects that harbor material containing infectious agent
11. Center for Medicare and Medicaid Services initials
13. Federal law that was designed to regulate patient privacy (abbrev.)
14. Code used to classify, report, and bill health care services
15. Pre-established value indicating a level of acceptable practice
16. College of American Pathologists initials
18. Compares a patient's current laboratory results with previous results for the same test
19. Global, nonprofit standards-developing organization
20. Intensive care unit for neonates
24. One of the barriers to communication
25. Type of isolation for a neutropenic patient
27. Level of care that should be exercised in the given circumstances
28. Abbreviation for hematocrit
30. Fluid found in the spinal column (abbrev.)
31. Infection acquired in a hospital
32. Tests that must be done immediately
33. Source of an infectious microorganism
34. An act or threat that causes one to be in fear of immediate battery
37. A process in which a party in a legal action is questioned under oath
39. Manufacturers must furnish this for hazardous products
40. Alanine aminotransferase (abbrev.)
41. Resistant to a particular disease or infection

DOWN

1. Antibody (abbrev.)
2. Educational standards for phlebotomy programs
4. Consent that implies voluntary and competent permission
5. AMT phlebotomy certification initials
6. Hospital advisory committee for infection-control (abbrev.)
8. Percutaneous exposure occurs through this type of skin
10. New initials for Clinical Laboratory Scientist (abbrev.)
12. Old initials for Clinical Laboratory Scientist (abbrev.)
17. Study of an individual's concept and use of space
19. Evidence that fundamental competencies in a particular field have been mastered
21. Means of transmission through food or water
22. Laboratory instrument that does urinalysis
23. Microbe capable of causing disease
24. Aspartate aminotransferase (abbrev.)
26. Microbes responsible for certain diseases such as the common cold
29. Personalized medicine abbreviation
31. Health professionals who give direct patient care
35. Blood types
36. Wrongful act against one's person
38. Chemical abbreviation for sodium

Chapter 4
Medical Terminology

Objectives

Study the information in your TEXTBOOK that corresponds to each objective to prepare yourself for the activities in this chapter.

1 Identify, define, and use basic word elements individually and within medical terms.

2 Demonstrate proper pronunciation of medical terms and unique plural endings.

3 Use common medical abbreviations and symbols and explain how items on the "Do Not Use" list can cause problems.

Matching

Use choices only once unless otherwise indicated.

MATCHING 4-1: KEY TERMS AND DESCRIPTIONS

Match each key term with the *best* description.

Key Terms (1–5)

1. _____ Combining form
2. _____ Combining vowel
3. _____ Prefix
4. _____ Suffix
5. _____ Word root

Descriptions

A. Comes before a word root and modifies its meaning
B. Establishes the basic meaning of a medical term
C. Follows a word root and adds to or changes the meaning
D. Identifies the plural form of a word
E. Makes pronunciation easier
F. Signifies a Latin word root
G. Word root joined with a vowel

MATCHING 4-2: WORD ROOTS AND MEANINGS

Match each word root with its meaning.

Word Roots

1. _____ chondr
2. _____ cry
3. _____ cyt
4. _____ derm
5. _____ glyc
6. _____ hemat
7. _____ lip
8. _____ leuk
9. _____ morph
10. _____ my
11. _____ sphygm
12. _____ squam
13. _____ thromb
14. _____ ren
15. _____ scler

Meanings

A. Bladder
B. Blood
C. Bone
D. Cartilage
E. Cell
F. Chest
G. Clot
H. Cold
I. Fat
J. Form
K. Hard
L. Kidney
M. Liver
N. Lung
O. Muscle
P. Pain
Q. Pulse
R. Scale
S. Skin
T. Sugar
U. White

MATCHING 4-3: PREFIXES AND MEANINGS

Match each prefix with its meaning.

Prefixes

1. _____ a-
2. _____ brady-
3. _____ dorso-
4. _____ epi-
5. _____ homeo-
6. _____ intra-
7. _____ macro-
8. _____ medi-
9. _____ neo-
10. _____ per-
11. _____ poly-
12. _____ tri-

Meanings

A. Back
B. Before
C. Between
D. Difficult
E. Equal
F. Large
G. Many
H. Middle
I. New
J. Outside
K. Over
L. Same
M. Slow
N. Three
O. Through
P. Unequal
Q. Within
R. Without

MATCHING 4-4: SUFFIXES AND MEANINGS

Match each suffix with its meaning.

Suffixes

1. _____ -algia
2. _____ -emia
3. _____ -ic
4. _____ -ism
5. _____ -itis
6. _____ -lysis
7. _____ -meter
8. _____ -oxia
9. _____ -penia
10. _____ -stasis
11. _____ -tomy
12. _____ -ule

Meanings

A. Blood condition
B. Breakdown
C. Burst forth
D. Condition
E. Deficiency
F. Incision
G. Infection
H. Inflammation
I. Measuring instrument
J. O_2 level
K. Pain
L. Pertaining to
M. Recording
N. Small
O. Specialist
P. Stopping
Q. Tumor
R. Twitch

Labeling Exercises

LABELING EXERCISE 4-1: WORD ELEMENTS AND MEANINGS

Identify the highlighted element in each medical term listed below. Write the type of element (prefix, word root, combining vowel or form, or suffix) and its meaning on the corresponding line. If the element has no meaning, write NA.

Medical Term	Type of Element	Element Meaning
1. arteriospasm	_____	_____
2. cyanotic	_____	_____
3. cytology	_____	_____
4. diapedesis	_____	_____
5. endocrinologist	_____	_____
6. hemopoiesis	_____	_____
7. neonatal	_____	_____
8. osteochondritis	_____	_____
9. postprandial	_____	_____
10. tachycardia	_____	_____

LABELING EXERCISE 4-2: SINGULAR AND PLURAL WORD ENDINGS

Highlight the word endings in each of the medical terms below and circle any that are plural. Write the applicable singular or plural form of the term on the corresponding line.

1. lumina _____

2. ova _____

3. papillae _____

4. phalanx _____

5. protozoa _____

LABELING EXERCISE 4-3: PRONUNCIATION GUIDELINES

1. Circle the terms below in which the "g" is pronounced like a "j."

   gallbladder/genetic/Giardia/gonad/gyrate

2. Circle the terms below in which the ending is pronounced like "eye."

   chordae/diastole/fungi/myalgia/nuclei

3. Circle the terms below in which the "c" is pronounced like an "s."

   Capillary/cell/circulation/colitis/cytology

4. Circle the terms below in which the "e" at the end is pronounced separately.

   Adipose/arteriole/diastole/exocrine/syncope

Knowledge Drills

KNOWLEDGE DRILL 4-1: KEY POINT RECOGNITION

The following sentences are taken from Key Point statements found in Chapter 4 of the textbook. Fill in the blanks with the missing information.

1. A (A) _____ _____ typically indicates a (B) _____, organ, body system, color, condition, substance, or (C) _____.

2. However, a combining (A) _____ is kept between two (B) _____ _____, even if the second (C) _____ (D) _____ begins with a vowel.

3. When a suffix begins with (A) _____, the (B) _____ is (C) _____ as in hemorrhage.

4. When a suffix is added to a word ending in (A) _____, the (B) _____ is changed to a (C) _____ or _____, as in pharynx becoming (D) _____ and (E) _____ becoming thoracic.

5. It is more important to be able to identify the (A) _____ of a word (B) _____ than to identify its (C) _____.

6. To determine the meaning of a medical term, it is generally best to start with the (A) _____, then go to the (B) _____, and identify the meaning of the (C) _____ _____ or (D) _____ last.

7. A (A) _____ (B) _____ is not normally used when a suffix starts with a (C) _____.

8. Occasionally there will be both a (A) _____ and (B) _____ word (C) _____ with the same meaning.

9. For example, the word root (A) _____ means "vein," a (B) _____ (C) _____.

10. When a (A) _____ begins with a vowel and the word (B) _____ ends in the same vowel, one is dropped as in (C) _____.

KNOWLEDGE DRILL 4-2: SCRAMBLED WORDS

Unscramble the following words using the hints given in parenthesis and the letters that have been placed in the correct boxes. Finish writing the correct spelling of the scrambled word in the corresponding box.

1. thagolpoy (the study of disease)

		t				o		

2. sloycligys (breakdown of sugar)

	l						s		

3. tecalanubit (pertaining to in front of the elbow)

		t				b				

4. tucubansouse (beneath the skin)

			c			a			u	

5. yendasp (difficult breathing)

	y				e	

6. nelra (pertaining to the kidneys)

	e		a	

7. vexalcasutrar (outside the blood vessels)

			r		a		u			

8. cetryocmi (a small cell)

			r				e	

9. trienesti (intestinal inflammation)

			e		i			

10. critocles (pertaining to being hard)

	c					t		

KNOWLEDGE DRILL 4-3: TRUE/FALSE ACTIVITY

1 to 10: The following statements are all false. Circle the one or two words that make the statement false and write the correct word(s) that would make the statement true, in the space provided.

1. The basic meaning of a medical term is defined by the suffix. _____

2. The prefix of the medical term *toxicology* is *toxi*. _____

3. The Greek root *nephr* and the Latin root *ren* both mean liver. _____

4. A suffix adds to the meaning of a prefix. _____

5. The word root of the medical term coronary means heart. _____

6. A word root combined with a prefix is called a combining form. _____

7. The suffix of the word hyperthyroidism means high. _____

8. The singular form of the word phalanges is phalange. _____

9. The meaning of the abbreviation NPO is nothing to drink. _____

10. The "e" in systole is silent. _____

11. Ilium means hip bone, and is pronounced the same as ileum, which means large intestine. _____
_____

12. The plural of ovum is ovae. _____

13. The prefix of the word exocrine means below. _____

14. The most common combining vowel is "a." _____

15. ESR is the abbreviation for erythrocyte sedimentation ratio. _____

Skills Drills

SKILLS DRILL 4-1: REQUISITION ACTIVITY

Any Hospital USA
1123 West Physician Drive
Any Town USA

Laboratory Test Requisition

- -

PATIENT INFORMATION:

Name: _____
(last)   (first)   (MI)

Identification Number: _____ Birth Date: _____

Referring Physician: _____

Date to be Collected: _____ Time to be Collected: _____

Special Instructions: _____

- -

TEST(S) REQUIRED:

ASO _____   Hgb _____
Bili _____   Lytes _____
CBC _____   O&P _____
Chol _____   PT _____
CK _____   PTT _____
DIC _____   RBC _____
ESR _____   RPR _____
FSH _____   TIBC _____
Gluc _____   TSH _____
GTT _____   UA _____

The following requisition contains abbreviations for common laboratory tests. Write the full name of the test in the space provided on the requisition.

SKILLS DRILL 4-2: WORD BUILDING

Build medical terms for each definition listed below. Identify each word element, prefix (P), word root (WR), combining vowel (CV), or suffix (S) needed to build the term and write the meaning of each element on the appropriate line.

1. blood tumor

   Elements _____ /_____
                         WR   S

2. cutting the vein

   Elements _____ /_____ /_____
                         WR   CV   S

3. low blood sugar

   Elements _____ /_____ /_____
                         P   WR   S

4. condition of death

   Elements _____ /_____
                         WR   S

5. inflammation of the liver

   Elements _____ /_____
                         WR   S

6. clotting cell

   Elements _____ /_____ /_____
                         WR   CV   S

7. specialist in the study of disease

   Elements _____ /_____ /_____
                         WR   CV   S

8. large cell

   Elements _____ /_____
                         P   S

9. stopping blood (or blood flow)

   Elements _____ /_____ /_____
                         WR   CV   S

10. pertaining to poison

    Elements _____ /_____
                          WR   S

11. study of tissue

    Elements _____ /_____
                          WR   S

12. pertaining to the head

    Elements _____ /_____
                          WR   S

13. condition of hard arteries

    Elements _____ /_____ /_____ /_____
                          WR   CV   WR   S

14. inflammation of the brain

    Elements _____ /_____
                          WR   S

15. pertaining to through the skin

    Elements _____ /_____ /_____
                          P   WR   S

Crossword

ACROSS

1. Prefix meaning different
3. Word root meaning glucose
5. Fasting blood sugar (abbrev.)
6. Prefix meaning small
9. Prefix meaning difficult
10. Before surgery (abbrev.)
11. Prefix meaning half
12. Word root meaning heart
15. Word root meaning vein
16. Prefix meaning below
17. Word root meaning intestines
18. Word root meaning clot
21. Word root meaning disease
22. Word root meaning kidney
23. Word root meaning head
27. Glucose tolerance test (abbrev.)
28. Word root meaning bone
30. Word root meaning tumor
31. Suffix meaning abnormal flow
33. Prefix meaning around
34. Word root meaning brain
37. Word root meaning chest
40. Word root meaning fiber
42. Prefix meaning within
43. Suffix meaning tumor
45. Prefix meaning after
46. Suffix meaning enzyme

DOWN

1. Prefix meaning same
2. Erythrocyte sedimentation rate (abbrev.)
3. Word root meaning stomach
4. Prefix meaning through
5. Fever of unknown origin (abbrev.)
7. Prefix meaning blue
8. Suffix meaning condition
9. Disseminated intravascular coagulation (abbrev.)
10. Word root meaning vein
13. Word root meaning joint
14. Word root meaning artery
19. Word root meaning kidney
20. Word root meaning liver
21. Word root meaning lung
24. Word root meaning air
25. Suffix meaning specialist in study of
26. Word root meaning vessel
27. Word root meaning sugar
29. Word root meaning hard
32. Combining form meaning blood
35. Word root meaning death
36. Prefix meaning against
38. Word root meaning bile
39. Suffix meaning inflammation
41. Prefix meaning new
44. Prefix meaning poor

Chapter Review Questions

1. This word element establishes the basic meaning of a medical term.
   - a. Combining form
   - b. Prefix
   - c. Suffix
   - d. Word root

2. Of the following word parts which is a prefix?
   - a. epi
   - b. gram
   - c. lip
   - d. ole

3. To what part of the body does the word cephal refer?
   - a. Kidney
   - b. Head
   - c. Intestine
   - d. Liver

4. Which part of the word pericarditis is the word root?
   - a. ardi
   - b. cardi
   - c. itis
   - d. peri

5. What does the suffix -lysis mean?
   - a. Breakdown
   - b. Incision
   - c. Stoppage
   - d. Surgical puncture

6. The plural form of ovum is
   - a. ova.
   - b. ovae.
   - c. ovi
   - d. ovix.

7. The singular form of atria is
   - a. atra.
   - b. atrius.
   - c. atrix.
   - d. atrium.

8. The medical term for platelet is
   - a. coagulocyte.
   - b. hepatocyte.
   - c. leukocyte.
   - d. thrombocyte.

9. Venule means
   - a. condition of a vein.
   - b. pertaining to a vein.
   - c. small vein.
   - d. vein tumor.

10. Which of the following means kidney inflammation?
    - a. Nephremia
    - b. Nephritis
    - c. Renemia
    - d. Renitis

11. The "e" at the end is pronounced separately in
    - a. arteriole.
    - b. flange.
    - c. syncope.
    - d. venule.

12. The abbreviation ESR stands for
    - a. erythrocyte sedimentation rate.
    - b. established secondary reaction.
    - c. estimated sedimentation range.
    - d. evaluated survival response.

13. The abbreviation RBC means
    - a. random blood count.
    - b. rare blood cancer.
    - c. red blood cell.
    - d. reduced blood content.

14. The abbreviation PPD means
    - a. platelet plasma donor.
    - b. postprandial diet.
    - c. potassium and phosphorus determination.
    - d. purified protein derivative.

15. Which of the following abbreviations is on the Joint Commission's current "Do Not Use" List?
    - a. ACTH
    - b. HbSAg
    - c. MSO_4
    - d. PCO_2

16. If a phlebotomy program decides to become nationally approved, it would contact which organization?
    - a. ASCLS
    - b. CLIA
    - c. DHS
    - d. NAACLS

17. The prefix of the word antiseptic means
    - a. against.
    - b. away from.
    - c. difficult.
    - d. without.

18. The law that was designed to make health insurance more portable and accountable is
    - a. ACA
    - b. ACO
    - c. HCFA
    - d. HIPAA

Case Studies

Case Study 4-1: Laboratory Orders

A phlebotomist receives a telephone order from the ICU requesting stat collection of ABGs, lytes, and a WBC on a patient with COPD.

QUESTIONS

1. What is the complete name of the patient's location?

2. What is the collection priority and what does it mean?

3. What are the complete names of the tests that the phlebotomist will collect?

4. What is the complete name of the disorder the patient has?

Case Study 4-2: Outpatient Blood Draw

A patient arrives at an outpatient surgery blood drawing station with a requisition from her physician for a pre-op CBC and a chem profile. The requisition indicates that the patient has h/o syncope and must be fasting for the tests and NPO for surgery, which is scheduled for later that morning.

QUESTIONS

1. Why is the patient having the blood tests?

2. What does NPO mean and how does the phlebotomist determine that the patient is NPO?

3. Look up the meaning of syncope in the glossary in the TEXTBOOK. What does h/o syncope mean? Should it concern the phlebotomist? Why or why not?

Case Study 4-3: Safety Issues and Gloving

A recent case of HBV in the laboratory suggests that there are safety issues and that OSHA standards are not being followed. The phlebotomist that became contaminated claims that the gloves they use in the laboratory are not quality and that is why she was exposed. Her supervisor tells her that the gloves are FDA certified and CAP inspections also verify the safety of the gloves.

QUESTIONS

1. Write the complete name of the disease that the phlebotomist contracted?

2. Spell out the name of the national organization that governs glove quality?

3. What is the complete name of the laboratory organization that inspects and accredits laboratories?

4. Write the complete name of the federal agency that sets safety standards for the laboratory?

Chapter 5

Human Anatomy and Physiology Review

Objectives

Study the information in your TEXTBOOK associated with each objective to prepare yourself for the activities in this chapter.

1 Demonstrate basic knowledge of the terminology, functions, and organization of the body.

2 Describe functions, identify components or major structures, and correctly use terminology associated with each body system.

3 List disorders and diagnostic tests commonly associated with each body system.

Matching

Use choices only once unless otherwise indicated.

MATCHING 5-1: KEY TERMS AND DESCRIPTIONS

Match each key term with the *best* description.

Key Terms (1–20)

1. _____ Acidosis
2. _____ Alkalosis
3. _____ Alveoli
4. _____ Anabolism
5. _____ Anatomical position
6. _____ Anatomy
7. _____ Anterior
8. _____ Avascular
9. _____ Axons
10. _____ Body cavities
11. _____ Body plane
12. _____ Bursae
13. _____ Cartilage
14. _____ Catabolism
15. _____ Diaphragm
16. _____ Distal
17. _____ Dorsal
18. _____ Endocrine glands
19. _____ Exocrine glands
20. _____ Frontal plane

Descriptions

A. Air sacs in the lungs where exchange of gases takes place
B. Breakdown of complex substances into simple ones
C. Condition that results from a decrease in the pH of body fluids
D. Condition that results from an increase in the pH of body fluids
E. Conversion of simple compounds into complex substances
F. Farthest from the point of attachment
G. Flat surface of a real or imaginary cut through the body
H. Glands that secrete substances directly into the bloodstream
I. Glands that secrete substances through ducts
J. Hollow body spaces that house body organs
K. Means "at the back of the body or body part"
L. Muscle that separates the thoracic and abdominal cavities
M. Nerve fibers that conduct impulses away from the nerve cell body
N. Real or imaginary cut that divides the body vertically into front and back portions
O. Referring to the front
P. Small synovial fluid–filled sacs found near joints
Q. Standing erect with arms at the side and eyes and palms facing forward
R. Study of the structural composition of living things
S. Type of hard, nonvascular connective tissue
T. Without blood or lymph vessels

Key Terms (21–40)

21. _____ Gametes
22. _____ Hemopoiesis
23. _____ Homeostasis
24. _____ Hormones
25. _____ Meninges
26. _____ Metabolism
27. _____ Mitosis
28. _____ Nephron
29. _____ Neuron
30. _____ Phalanges

Descriptions

A. Balanced or steady state
B. Chemical substances that affect many body processes
C. Connective tissue that encloses the brain and spinal chord
D. Divides the body horizontally into upper and lower portions
E. Divides the body vertically into right and left portions
F. Finger bones
G. Functional unit of the kidney
H. Fundamental unit of the nervous system
I. Gland secreting hormones that control other glands
J. Has the same meaning as anterior
K. Joint fluid
L. Lying face down and the act of turning face down
M. Lying face up and the act of turning face up
N. Nearest to the point of attachment
O. Process by which cells divide

31. _____ Physiology

32. _____ Pituitary gland

33. _____ Prone/pronation

34. _____ Proximal

35. _____ Sagittal plane

36. _____ Supine/supination

37. _____ Surfactant

38. _____ Synovial fluid

39. _____ Transverse plane

40. _____ Ventral

P. Production of blood cells
Q. Sex cells
R. Study of the function of living things
S. Substance that coats the alveoli
T. Sum of all physical and chemical reactions that sustain life

MATCHING 5-2: STRUCTURES, DISORDERS, DIAGNOSTIC TESTS, AND BODY SYSTEMS

Match the structures, disorders, and diagnostic tests with the appropriate body systems. Choices may be used more than once.

Structures

1. _____ Biceps

2. _____ Bronchus

3. _____ Calcaneus

4. _____ Dendrite

5. _____ Esophagus

6. _____ Fallopian tube

7. _____ Glomerulus

8. _____ Papilla

9. _____ Sebaceous gland

10. _____ Thymus

Disorders

1. _____ Atrophy

2. _____ Bursitis

3. _____ Dermatitis

4. _____ Diabetes mellitus

5. _____ Emphysema

6. _____ Hepatitis

7. _____ Hypothyroidism

8. _____ Meningitis

9. _____ Nephritis

10. _____ Prostate cancer

Diagnostic Tests

1. _____ AFB culture

2. _____ Bilirubin

3. _____ CSF analysis

4. _____ Creatine kinase

5. _____ Creatinine clearance

6. _____ Skin scraping KOH prep

7. _____ O & P

8. _____ RPR

9. _____ TSH

10. _____ Uric acid

Body Systems

A. Digestive
B. Endocrine
C. Muscular
D. Nervous
E. Integumentary
F. Reproductive
G. Respiratory
H. Skeletal
I. Urinary

Labeling Exercises

LABELING EXERCISE 5-1: BODY PLANES (Text Fig. 5-1)

1. Write the names of the three body planes on the correct numbered lines in different colors.
2. Color each plane in the illustration with the color used to write the name.

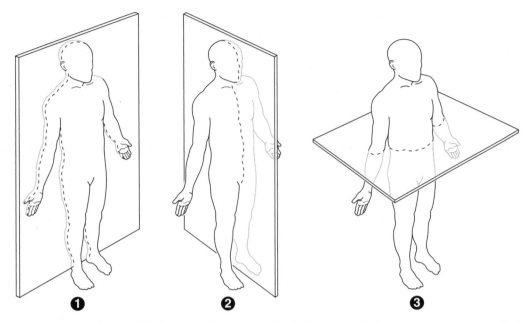

(Adapted with permission from BJ Cohen, KL Hull. *Study Guide for Memmler's the Human Body in Health and Disease*, 12th ed. Philadelphia: Lippincott Williams & Wilkins; 2013:7.)

1. _____

2. _____

3. _____

LABELING EXERCISE 5-2: DIRECTIONAL TERMS (Text Fig. 5-2)

1. Write the name of each directional term on the numbered lines in different colors.
2. Color the arrow corresponding to each directional term with the color used to write the name.

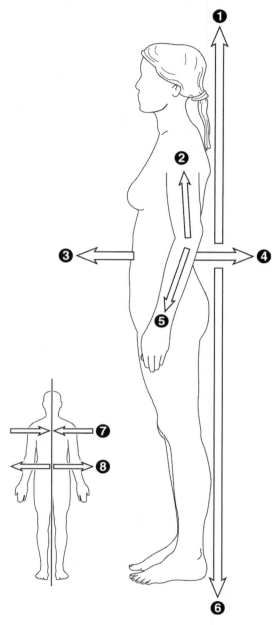

(Adapted with permission from BJ Cohen, KL Hull. *Study Guide for Memmler's the Human Body in Health and Disease*, 12th ed. Philadelphia: Lippincott Williams & Wilkins: 2013:6.)

1. _____

2. _____

3. _____

4. _____

5. _____

6. _____

7. _____

8. _____

LABELING EXERCISE 5-3: LATERAL VIEW OF BODY CAVITIES (Text Fig. 5-3)

1. Identify the numbered body cavities and other structures and write the names on the corresponding lines below using different colors for each one.
2. Color each cavity or structure with the color used to write the name.

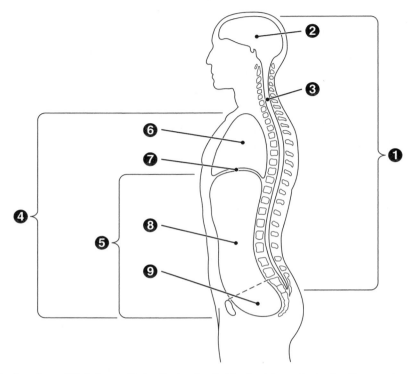

(Adapted with permission from BJ Cohen, KL Hull. *Study Guide for Memmler's the Human Body in Health and Disease*, 12th ed. Philadelphia: Lippincott Williams & Wilkins: 2013:8.)

1. _____   6. _____

2. _____   7. _____

3. _____   8. _____

4. _____   9. _____

5. _____

LABELING EXERCISE 5-4: CELL DIAGRAM (Text Fig. 5-4)

1. Write the names of the numbered structures in different colors on the corresponding lines.
2. Color each numbered structure with the color used to write the name.

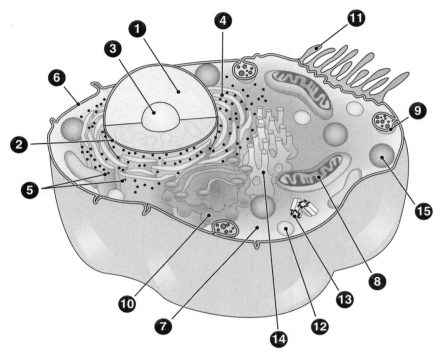

(Adapted with permission from BJ Cohen, KL Hull. *Study Guide for Memmler's the Human Body in Health and Disease*, 12th ed. Philadelphia: Lippincott Williams & Wilkins; 2012:41.)

1. _____
2. _____
3. _____
4. _____
5. _____
6. _____
7. _____
8. _____

9. _____
10. _____
11. _____
12. _____
13. _____
14. _____
15. _____

LABELING EXERCISE 5-5: INTEGUMENTARY SYSTEM (Text Fig. 5-5)

1. Identify the skin layers shown in numbers 1 through 3 and write the names in the corresponding boxes.
2. Use different colors to write the names of the other numbered structures on the corresponding lines below. Use red if the structure is an artery; blue if it is a vein; and yellow if it is a nerve.
3. Color the various structures within the diagram with the color used to write the name. Remember, some structures are found in more than one place.

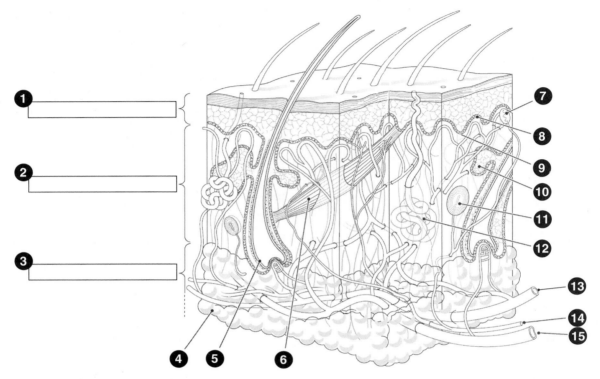

(Adapted with permission from BJ Cohen, KL Hull. *Study Guide for Memmler's the Human Body in Health and Disease*, 12th ed. Philadelphia: Lippincott Williams & Wilkins; 2013:98.)

4. _____   11. _____

5. _____   12. _____

6. _____   13. _____

7. _____   14. _____

8. _____   15. _____

9. _____

10. _____

LABELING EXERCISE 5-6: MUSCULAR SYSTEM (Text Fig. 5-7)

1. Write the names of the three types of muscle tissue in the appropriate blanks using different colors.
2. Color the muscle cells in the corresponding illustration color used to write the name. Color the nuclei a different color. Use the same nuclei color for all three illustrations.
3. Draw an arrow from appropriate muscle illustration to the corresponding site on the body.

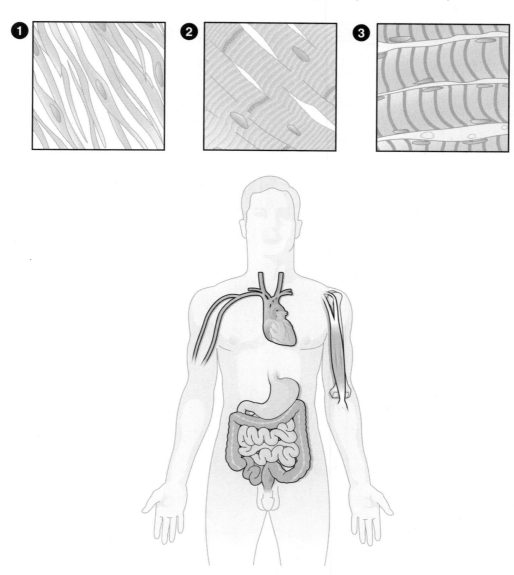

(Adapted with permission from BJ Cohen, KL Hull. *Study Guide for Memmler's the Human Body in Health and Disease*, 12th ed. Philadelphia: Lippincott Williams & Wilkins; 2013:58.)

1. _____

2. _____

3. _____

LABELING EXERCISE 5-7: HUMAN SKELETON (Text Fig. 5-8)

1. Write the name of each labeled part on the numbered lines in different colors. Use the same color for structures 19 and 20 and structures 23 to 25.
2. Color the different structures on the diagram with the color used to write the name. Try to color every structure in the figure with the appropriate color. For instance, structure number 3 is found in two locations.

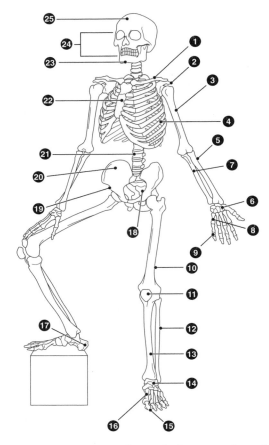

(Adapted with permission from BJ Cohen, KL Hull. *Study Guide for Memmler's the Human Body in Health and Disease*, 12th ed. Philadelphia: Lippincott Williams & Wilkins; 2013:124.)

1. _____
2. _____
3. _____
4. _____
5. _____
6. _____
7. _____
8. _____
9. _____
10. _____
11. _____
12. _____
13. _____

14. _____
15. _____
16. _____
17. _____
18. _____
19. _____
20. _____
21. _____
22. _____
23. _____
24. _____
25. _____

LABELING EXERCISE 5-8: NERVOUS SYSTEM (Text Fig. 5-9)

1. Identify the numbered parts and divisions of the nervous system and write the names on the corresponding lines below.
2. Color the central nervous system structures yellow and the visible peripheral nervous system structures green.

Posterior view

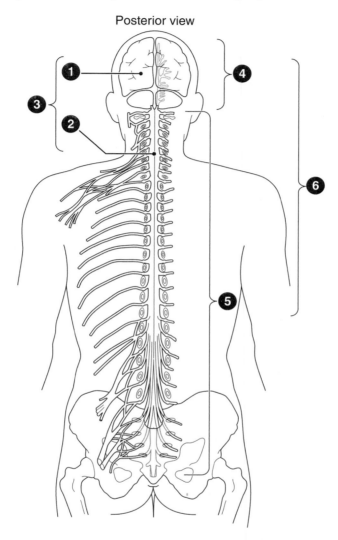

(Adapted with permission from BJ Cohen, KL Hull. *Study Guide for Memmler's the Human Body in Health and Disease*, 12th ed. Philadelphia: Lippincott Williams & Wilkins; 2013:169.)

1. _____   4. _____
2. _____   5. _____
3. _____   6. _____

LABELING EXERCISE 5-9: MOTOR NEURON (Text Fig. 5-10)

1. Use different colors to write the names of the numbered structures on the corresponding lines below.
2. Color the structures within the diagram the same colors used to write their names. Do not color structures 5 and 6.
3. Add large arrows to the diagram showing the direction the nerve impulse will travel to get from the dendrites to the muscle.

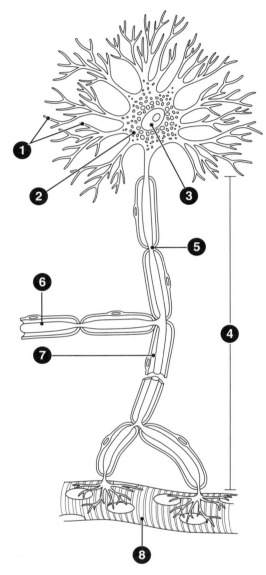

(Adapted with permission from BJ Cohen, KL Hull. *Study Guide for Memmler's the Human Body in Health and Disease*, 12th ed. Philadelphia: Lippincott Williams & Wilkins; 2013:170.)

1. _____   5. _____

2. _____   6. _____

3. _____   7. _____

4. _____   8. _____

LABELING EXERCISE 5-10: ENDOCRINE SYSTEM (Text Fig. 5-11)

1. Use different colors to write the names of the numbered structures on the corresponding lines below.
2. Color the structures within the diagram the color used to write the name. Some structures are present in more than one location. Color all of a particular structure the appropriate color. For instance, color or outline all three parathyroid glands, although only one is numbered.

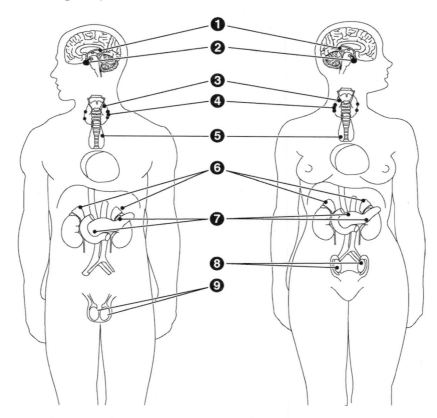

(Adapted with permission from BJ Cohen, KL Hull. *Study Guide for Memmler's the Human Body in Health and Disease*, 12th ed. Philadelphia: Lippincott Williams & Wilkins; 2013:230.)

1. _____   6. _____

2. _____   7. _____

3. _____   8. _____

4. _____   9. _____

5. _____

LABELING EXERCISE 5-11: DIGESTIVE SYSTEM (Text Fig. 5-12)

1. Trace the path of food through the digestive tract by writing the names of the structures numbered 1 through 12 on the corresponding lines. Color all of these structures orange.
2. Write the names of the accessory organs and ducts on the appropriate lines in different colors. Use black for structure 18.
3. Color each accessory organ with the color used to write its name.

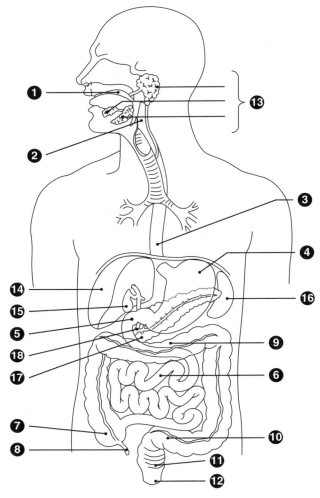

(Adapted with permission from BJ Cohen, KL Hull. *Study Guide for Memmler's the Human Body in Health and Disease*, 12th ed. Philadelphia: Lippincott Williams & Wilkins; 2013:363.)

1. _____
2. _____
3. _____
4. _____
5. _____
6. _____
7. _____
8. _____
9. _____

10. _____
11. _____
12. _____
13. _____
14. _____
15. _____
16. _____
17. _____
18. _____

LABELING EXERCISE 5-12: MALE REPRODUCTIVE SYSTEM (Text Fig. 5-13A)

1. Write the names of the numbered structures of the male reproductive systems in different colors on the corresponding lines below. Use the same color for structures 1 and 12.
2. Color the structures within the diagrams the colors used to write their names.

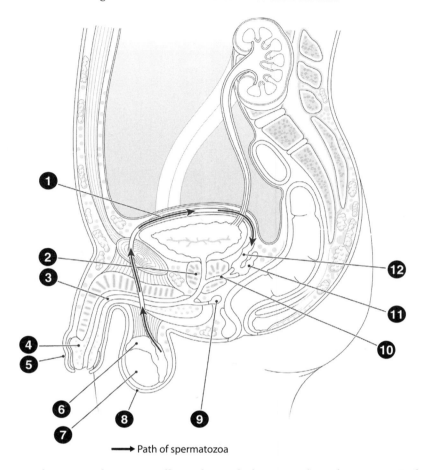

→ Path of spermatozoa

(Adapted with permission from BJ Cohen, KL Hull. *Study Guide for Memmler's the Human Body in Health and Disease*, 12th ed. Philadelphia: Lippincott Williams & Wilkins; 2013:432.)

1. _____   7. _____

2. _____   8. _____

3. _____   9. _____

4. _____   10. _____

5. _____   11. _____

6. _____   12. _____

LABELING EXERCISE 5-13: FEMALE REPRODUCTIVE SYSTEM (Text Fig. 5-13B)

1. Write the names of the numbered structures of the female reproductive systems in different colors on the corresponding lines below.
2. Color the structures within the diagrams the colors used to write their names.

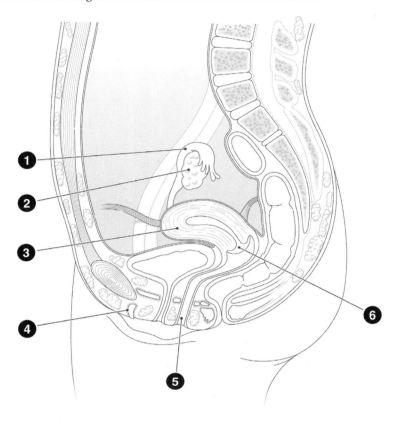

(Adapted with permission from BJ Cohen, KL Hull. *Study Guide for Memmler's the Human Body in Health and Disease*, 12th ed. Philadelphia: Lippincott Williams & Wilkins; 2013:438.)

1. _____   4. _____

2. _____   5. _____

3. _____   6. _____

LABELING EXERCISE 5-14: URINARY SYSTEM (MALE) (Text Fig. 5-14)

1. Write the names of the numbered structures on the corresponding lines below using different colors. Use red for arteries and blue for veins.
2. Color the structures within the diagram colors used to write the names.
3. Write the name of the functional unit of the kidney on line 8.
4. Write the name of the filtering tufts of capillaries within the kidney on line 9.

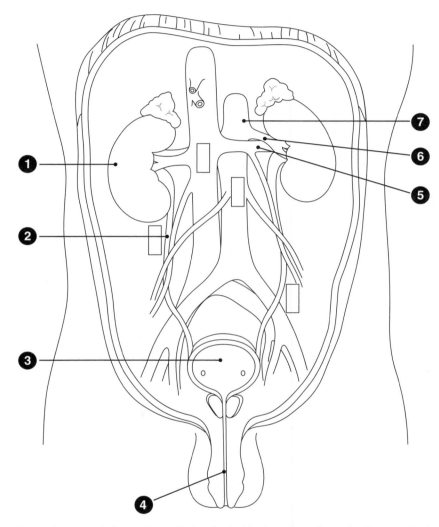

(Adapted with permission from BJ Cohen, KL Hull. *Study Guide for Memmler's the Human Body in Health and Disease*, 12th ed. Philadelphia: Lippincott Williams & Wilkins; 2013:406.)

1. _____   6. _____

2. _____   7. _____

3. _____   8. _____

4. _____   9. _____

5. _____

LABELING EXERCISE 5-15: RESPIRATORY SYSTEM (Text Fig. 5-15)

1. Write the names of the numbered structures on the corresponding lines below.
2. Color all of the structures in the main illustration that encounter inspired air green.

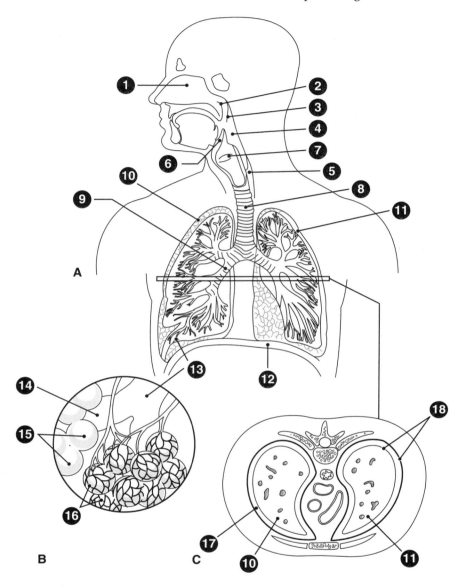

(Adapted with permission from BJ Cohen, KL Hull. *Study Guide for Memmler's the Human Body in Health and Disease*, 12th ed. Philadelphia: Lippincott Williams & Wilkins; 2013:340.)

1. _____
2. _____
3. _____
4. _____
5. _____
6. _____
7. _____
8. _____
9. _____

10. _____
11. _____
12. _____
13. _____
14. _____
15. _____
16. _____
17. _____
18. _____

Knowledge Drills

KNOWLEDGE DRILL 5-1: KEY POINT RECOGNITION

The following sentences are taken from Key Point statements found in Chapter 5 of the TEXTBOOK. Fill in the blanks with the missing information.

1. Blood creatinine is a measure of kidney function because (A) _____ is a (B) _____ product normally removed from the blood by the (C) _____ _____ _____ (_____).

2. Pregnancy tests are based on a reaction with a hormone called (A) _____ secreted by (B) _____ cells that eventually give rise to the (C) _____.

3. (A) _____ terms are relative positions in respect to other parts of the body. For example, the ankle can be described as (B) _____ to the leg and (C) _____ to the foot.

4. Bones of particular importance in capillary blood collection are the distal (A) _____ of the (B) _____ and the (C) _____ or (D) _____ bone of the foot.

5. A deficiency of (A) _____ in premature infants causes the (B) _____ to collapse leading to a condition called (C) _____ _____ _____ _____.

6. When a typical cell duplicates itself, the (A) _____ doubles and the cell (B) _____ by a process called (C) _____.

7. Skeletal muscle (A) _____ helps keep blood moving through your (B) _____. For example, moving your (C) _____ helps move blood from your fingertips back to your (D) _____.

8. The (A) _____ cavity is separated from the (B) _____ cavity by a muscle called the (C) _____.

9. Two chromosomes called (A) _____ and (B) _____ determine gender. Every egg contains an (C) _____ chromosome.

10. Every sperm contains either an (A) _____ or a _____ chromosome. If an egg is fertilized by a sperm containing a (B) _____ the (C) _____ combination will result in a male fetus.

KNOWLEDGE DRILL 5-2: SCRAMBLED WORDS

Unscramble the following words using the hints given in parenthesis and the letters that have been placed in the correct boxes. Finish writing the correct spelling of the scrambled word in the corresponding box.

1. tralenxe (near the surface)

	x		e				

2. biosmanla (constructive process)

		a						m

3. ratgelaic (connective tissue)

c								e

4. haxplan (a short bone)

		a		a		

5. lekestla (type of muscle)

	k	e					

6. clanuggo (stimulates the liver)

		u				o	

7. gemsenin (a problem if inflamed)

		n		n			

8. yasleam (aids in digestion)

		y			s	

9. tageem (could end up a human)

				t	e	

10. tranufscat (lungs need it)

	u		f						

KNOWLEDGE DRILL 5-3: TRUE/FALSE ACTIVITY

The following statements are all false. Circle the one or two words that make the statement false and write the correct word(s) that would make the statement true in the space provided.

1. The main structures of the urinary system are two kidneys, one ureter, a urinary bladder and a urethra. _____

2. Ventral cavities are located in back of the body. _____

3. The balanced or "steady state" condition in the human body is called hemopoiesis. _____

4. Medial means toward the middle of the body and lateral means toward the back of the body. _____
   _____

5. Cytoplasm is the command center of the cell that contains the chromosomes or genetic material.
   _____

6. Examples of flat bones are wrist and ankle bones. _____

7. The skin and accessory structures within it form the Muscular System. _____

8. The dermis is the outermost and thinnest layer of the skin. _____

9. The subcutaneous layer of the skin is composed of connective and elastic tissue that connects the skin to the surface muscles. _____

10. The digestive system components form a continuous passageway starting at the stomach and going to the anus. _____

Skills Drills

SKILLS DRILL 5-1: REQUISITION ACTIVITY

Identify one body system associated with each of the tests ordered on the requisition below. Write the test abbreviations (if applicable) and the associated body systems on the following lines in the order the tests appear on the requisition starting with the left column.

Any Hospital USA
1123 West Physician Drive
Any Town USA

Laboratory Test Requisition

- -

PATIENT INFORMATION:

Name: ___Doe_____ ___John_____ _C_ DOB: ___12-05-52____
       (last)   (first)   (MI)

Identification Number: __0673519285_____ Location: __302B_____

Referring Physician: __Martinez_____

Date to be Collected: __05/09/2015_____ Time to be Collected: __0600____

Special Instructions: __fasting_____

- -

TEST(S) REQUIRED:

_____ NH4 – Ammonia	_____ Hgb – hemoglobin
_____ Bili – Bilirubin, total & direct	_____ Lact – lactic acid/lactate
_____ BMP – basic metabolic panel	_X_ Lytes – electrolytes
_____ BUN – Blood urea nitrogen	_____ Plt. Ct. – platelet count
_____ CBC – complete blood count	_X_ PSA – prostate specific antigen
_X_ Chol – cholesterol	_____ PT – prothrombin time
_____ D–dimer	_____ PTT – partial thromboplastin time
_____ ESR – erythrocyte sed rate	_____ RPR – rapid plasma reagin
_____ ETOH – alcohol	_X_ UA – Urinalysis
_____ Gluc – glucose	Other __TSH & Uric Acid_____

---

1. _____

2. _____

3. _____

4. _____

5. _____

6. _____

SKILLS DRILL 5-2: WORD BUILDING

Divide each word into all of its elements: preface (P), word root (WR), combining vowel (CV), and suffix (S). Write the word part and its definition on the corresponding lines. Write the general meaning of the word in the space provided. If the word does not have a particular word part, write NA (not applicable) in its place.

Example: Hyperglycemia

Elements _____*hyper*_____ / _____*glyc*_____ / ____*NA*____ / ____*emia*____
                              P   WR   CV   S

Definitions ____*too much*____ / ____*glucose*____ / _____ / _*blood condition*_

Meaning: a condition in which the blood sugar/glucose is high

1. Osteochondritis

   Elements _____ / _____ / _____ / _____
                   P   WR   CV   S

   Definitions _____ / _____ / _____ / _____

   Meaning:

2. Electromyogram _____ / _____ / _____ / _____
                                   P   WR   CV   S

   Definitions _____ / _____ / _____ / _____

   Meaning:

3. Physiology _____ / _____ / _____ / _____
                             P   WR   CV   S

   Definitions _____ / _____ / _____ / _____

   Meaning:

4. Thrombophlebitis _____ / _____ / _____ / _____
                                    P   WR   CV   S

   Definitions _____ / _____ / _____ / _____

   Meaning:

5. Dermatitis _____ / _____ / _____ / _____
                           P   WR   CV   S

   Definitions _____ / _____ / _____ / _____

   Meaning:

6. Arthritis _____ / _____ / _____ / _____
                        P   WR   CV   S

   Definitions _____ / _____ / _____ / _____

   Meaning:

Crossword

ACROSS

1. Act of turning the palm face up
4. Small synovial fluid–filled sacs near joints
6. O_2 and CO_2 form when disassociated from Hgb
7. Farthest from center of the body or point of attachment
8. Science of the functions of living organisms
10. Threadlike fiber carrying messages away from a nerve cell
11. Glands that secrete substances through ducts
13. Lateral, forearm bone
14. Sex cells
17. True skin
20. Medial forearm bone
21. Female reproductive gland containing ova
22. Large medial bone of the leg below the knee
23. Fundamental working unit of the nervous system
24. Aggregate of similar cells or types of cells
25. Multiple sclerosis (abbrev.)
26. Arterial blood gas procedure (abbrev.)
27. Dense connective tissue that makes up the skeletal system (pl.)
30. Concerning the palm of the hand
31. Intravenous pyelography (abbrev.)
33. Digestive system disorder that exhibits as a lesion
34. Largest accessory organ in the digestive system
36. A chronic lung disorder where exhaled air is obstructed (abbrev.)
37. Pancreatic disorder involving insulin
38. Nonliving material primarily composed of keratin

DOWN

1. Plane dividing the body into right and left portions
2. Nervous system division serving the body periphery (abbrev.)
3. Convoluted tubular structure in the kidney
4. Material part of a human described as head, neck, trunk, and limbs
5. Body process that converts simple compounds to complex substances
9. Substance that coats the wall of alveoli
12. Outside the blood vessels
15. Fibrous tissue that replaces normal tissue destroyed by injury
16. Hormone secreted by beta cells in the islets of Langerhans
18. Female hormone that stimulates secondary sex characteristics
19. Broad, flaring portion of the hip bone
26. Gland on top of each kidney
27. Fluid secreted by the liver that aids digestion of fat
28. Test that monitors joint swelling (abbrev.)
29. Bean-shaped organ located at the back of abdominal cavity
32. Test used to diagnose cervical cancer
35. Test that records brain waves (abbrev.)

Chapter Review Questions

1. The functional units of the nervous system are the
   - a. axons.
   - b. dendrites.
   - c. nephrons.
   - d. neurons.

2. A person who is supine is
   - a. lying face up.
   - b. lying on the side.
   - c. sitting up.
   - d. standing erect.

3. The creation of a hormone is an example of
   - a. anabolism.
   - b. catabolism.
   - c. hemopoiesis.
   - d. homeostasis.

4. Which of the following is a structure within a cell?
   - a. Alveolus
   - b. Glomerulus
   - c. Golgi apparatus
   - d. Pharynx

5. Which of the following is a finger bone?
   - a. Calcaneus
   - b. Phalanx
   - c. Tarsal
   - d. Tibia

6. Which of the following is an appendage of the integumentary system?
   - a. Adrenal gland
   - b. Pineal gland
   - c. Sebaceous gland
   - d. Thymus gland

7. A patient has meningitis. What body system is associated with this diagnosis?
   - a. Digestive
   - b. Endocrine
   - c. Nervous
   - d. Urinary

8. Which of the following are urinary system structures?
   - a. Meninges
   - b. Glomeruli
   - c. Islets of Langerhans
   - d. Papillae

9. Accessory organs of the digestive system include
   - a. the gallbladder.
   - b. the liver.
   - c. the pancreas.
   - d. all of the above.

10. Which of the following are all endocrine system tests?
    - a. ABGs, CBC, lytes
    - b. CBC, ESR, uric acid
    - c. FSH, HCG, RPR
    - d. T_3, T_4, TSH

11. Most carbon dioxide is carried in the blood in this manner.
    - a. As bicarbonate ion
    - b. As Pco_2
    - c. Bound to hemoglobin
    - d. Dissolved in the blood plasma

12. You are looking at muscle tissue under the microscope. The cells you see are long, cylindrical, multinucleated, and heavily striated. What type of muscle cells are they?
    - a. Cardiac
    - b. Involuntary
    - c. Smooth
    - d. Skeletal

13. Gametes are
    - a. blood-filtering structures.
    - b. cytoplasmic organelles.
    - c. dermal structures.
    - d. sex cells.

14. Surfactant
    - a. helps keep alveoli inflated.
    - b. is secreted by sebaceous glands.
    - c. is a digestive enzyme.
    - d. lubricates joints.

15. Which of the following tests is associated with the reproductive system?
    - a. ABG
    - b. HCG
    - c. O&P
    - d. UA

Case Studies

Case Study 5-1: Body Systems, Disorders, and Directional Terms

An elderly female outpatient arrives for a blood draw. The tests requested include ESR and estrogen levels. The patient walks in very slowly, as if her joints are stiff or sore. She has an oxygen tank with her. By the time she sits down in the chair, she is out of breath. When the phlebotomist attempts to locate a vein for the blood draw, the patient can only partly straighten her right arm and indicates that it is too painful to straighten it any further. The patient says that she cannot be drawn in the other arm because she has had a mastectomy on that side. The phlebotomist chooses a prominent vein on the medial aspect of the ventral surface of the arm slightly distal to the bend in the elbow to perform the blood draw.

QUESTIONS

1. Which of the patient's body systems are being evaluated at this time?

2. Name several disorders the patient could have based on her symptoms.

3. Where did the phlebotomist collect the specimen?

Case Study 5-2: Body Systems, Disorders, Diagnostic Tests, and Directional Terms

A phlebotomist is called to the ER to collect ABGs on a patient. The patient is highly agitated and hyperventilating. The phlebotomist collects the ABG specimen from an artery on the lateral aspect of the left ventral wrist proximal to the crease in the wrist.

QUESTIONS

1. What does the abbreviation ABG stand for?

2. What body system is evaluated with the ABG test?

3. What effect does hyperventilation have on CO_2 levels and pH?

4. What dangerous condition can hyperventilation cause?

5. Where did the phlebotomist collect the specimen?

Case Study 5-3: Outpatient in Wheelchair

A fragile male arrives at the outpatient draw station in a wheelchair and does not want to be moved to the phlebotomy chair because his right foot is too painful to stand on. The phlebotomist has drawn patients in this position before but is concerned in this case because this patient's arms have decreased muscle tissue, and he explains that his arms are almost too painful to touch. The area on the right arm proximal to wrist on the dorsal surface has a large vein, and the phlebotomist proceeds to carefully collect a uric acid, creatine kinase, and myoglobin from that site.

QUESTIONS

1. Which of the body systems are involved in this patient's condition?

2. Why is a uric acid test ordered?

3. What is the medical term for decreased muscle tissue?

4. What is the medical term for painful muscles?

5. Where did the phlebotomist collect the specimens?

Chapter 6

The Circulatory System

Objectives

Study the information in your TEXTBOOK that corresponds to each objective to prepare yourself for the activities in this chapter.

1   Demonstrate basic knowledge of the terminology, structures, functions, organization, and processes of the circulatory system.

2   Discuss the cardiac cycle, how an ECG tracing relates to it; the origins of heart sounds and pulse rates; and how to take and interpret blood pressure readings.

3   Distinguish between the different types of blood vessels and blood components, describe the structure and function of each, identify blood types and explain their importance, and trace the flow of blood throughout the circulatory system.

4   Name and locate major arm and leg veins and evaluate the suitability of each for venipuncture.

5   List the disorders and diagnostic tests of the circulatory system.

Matching

Use choices only once unless otherwise indicated.

MATCHING 6-1: KEY TERMS AND DESCRIPTIONS

Match the key term with the *best* description.

Key Terms (1–14)

1. _____ Antecubital
2. _____ Arrhythmia
3. _____ Atria
4. _____ Basilic vein
5. _____ Blood pressure
6. _____ Cardiac cycle
7. _____ Cephalic vein
8. _____ Coagulation
9. _____ Cross-match
10. _____ Diastole
11. _____ ECG/EKG
12. _____ Erythrocyte
13. _____ Extrinsic
14. _____ Fibrinolysis

Descriptions

A. Antecubital vein in the lateral aspect of the arm
B. Blood-clotting process
C. Force exerted by the blood on the walls of the blood vessels
D. Irregularity in the heart rate, rhythm, or beat
E. Large antecubital vein on the inner side of the arm
F. Medical term for red blood cell (RBC)
G. Medical term meaning in front of the elbow
H. One complete contraction and subsequent relaxation of the heart
I. Originating outside
J. Process that leads to dissolution of a blood clot
K. Record of the electrical activity of the heart
L. Relaxing phase of the cardiac cycle
M. Test to determine compatibility of blood for transfusion
N. Upper, receiving chambers of the heart

Key Terms (15–28)

15. _____ Hemostasis
16. _____ Intrinsic
17. _____ Leukocyte
18. _____ Median cubital vein
19. _____ Plasma
20. _____ Pulmonary circulation
21. _____ Serum
22. _____ Sphygmomanometer
23. _____ Systemic circulation
24. _____ Systole
25. _____ Thrombin
26. _____ Thrombocyte
27. _____ Vasoconstriction
28. _____ Ventricles

Descriptions

A. Blood pressure cuff
B. Contracting phase of the cardiac cycle
C. Fluid portion of clotted blood
D. Fluid portion of whole blood
E. Lower chambers of the heart, which deliver blood to the arteries
F. Main coagulation enzyme
G. Medical term for platelet
H. Medical term for white blood cell (WBC)
I. Originating within
J. Process by which the body stops blood loss after injury
K. Reduction in blood vessel diameter due to contraction of tunica media muscles
L. System that carries blood from the heart to the body tissues and back
M. System that carries blood from the heart to the lungs and back
N. Vein located near the middle of the antecubital fossa area

MATCHING 6-2: CIRCULATORY SYSTEM STRUCTURES, DISORDERS, AND DIAGNOSTIC TESTS

Match the structures, disorders, and diagnostic tests with the circulatory system components with which they are associated in the textbook using the following letters:

A (Blood); B (Heart); C (Lymphatic system); D (Vascular system)

Structures	**Disorders**	**Diagnostic Tests**
1. _____ Atria	1. _____ Anemia	1. _____ ABGs
2. _____ Axillary node	2. _____ Angina pectoris	2. _____ CBC
3. _____ Endocardium	3. _____ Atherosclerosis	3. _____ CK
4. _____ Eosinophil	4. _____ Endocarditis	4. _____ D-dimer
5. _____ Median vein	5. _____ Hodgkin disease	5. _____ Digoxin
6. _____ Reticulocyte	6. _____ Lymphoma	6. _____ Ferritin
7. _____ Septum	7. _____ Myocardial infarction	7. _____ Hgb
8. _____ Thoracic duct	8. _____ Phlebitis	8. _____ Mono test
9. _____ Tricuspid valve	9. _____ Polycythemia	9. _____ PT
10. _____ Tunica media	10. _____ Thrombocytopenia	10. _____ Troponin

MATCHING 6-3: HEMOSTATIC RESPONSE AND ACTION

Match the hemostatic response with the correct action. Choices may be used more than once.

Hemostatic Response

A. Vasoconstriction
B. Platelet plug formation
C. Hemostatic plug formation
D. Fibrinolysis

Action

1. _____ Amplification

2. _____ Blood vessel contraction

3. _____ Cross-linkage of fibrin

4. _____ Initiation

5. _____ Fibrin degradation

6. _____ Platelet adhesion

7. _____ Propagation

8. _____ Soluble fibrin generation

9. _____ Thrombin burst

10. _____ Tissue factor activation

Labeling Exercises

LABELING EXERCISE 6-1: THE HEART AND GREAT VESSELS (Text Fig. 6-1)

1. Write the name of each numbered structure on the corresponding numbered line.
2. Write the names of hollow spaces and vessels that contain deoxygenated blood in blue and those that contain oxygenated blood in red. Write the names of all other structures in black.
3. Color the layers and partition of the heart pink, the valves yellow, the vessels and structures that carry deoxygenated blood blue, and the vessels and structures that carry oxygenated blood red.
4. Draw arrows to indicate the direction of blood flow.

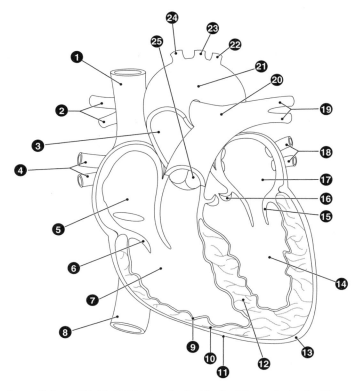

(Adapted with permission from Cohen BJ, Hull KL. *Study Guide for Memmler's the Human Body in Health and Disease,* 12th ed. Philadelphia: Lippincott Williams & Wilkins; 2013:268.)

1. _____   14. _____

2. _____   15. _____

3. _____   16. _____

4. _____   17. _____

5. _____   18. _____

6. _____   19. _____

7. _____   20. _____

8. _____   21. _____

9. _____   22. _____

10. _____   23. _____

11. _____   24. _____

12. _____   25. _____

13. _____

LABELING EXERCISE 6-2: ELECTRICAL CONDUCTION SYSTEM OF THE HEART (Text Fig. 6-2)

1. Write the name of each numbered structure of the electrical conduction system on the corresponding numbered line. Write the names of hollow spaces and vessels that contain deoxygenated blood in blue and those that contain oxygenated blood in red.
2. Color the structures that conduct electrical impulses yellow. Color the vessels and structures that carry deoxygenated blood blue and those that carry oxygenated blood red.
3. Place a star on the drawing next to the number of the structure that originates the electrical impulse.

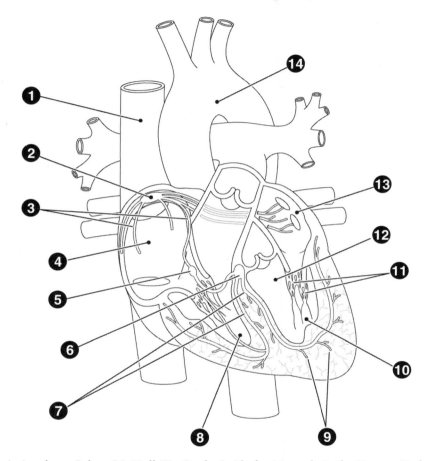

(Adapted with permission from Cohen BJ, Hull KL. *Study Guide for Memmler's the Human Body in Health and Disease,* 12th ed. Philadelphia: Lippincott Williams & Wilkins; 2013:271.)

1. _____

2. _____

3. _____

4. _____

5. _____

6. _____

7. _____

8. _____

9. _____

10. _____

11. _____

12. _____

13. _____

14. _____

LABELING EXERCISE 6-3: ARTERY, VEIN, AND CAPILLARY STRUCTURE (Text Fig. 6-8)

1. Write the names of the vessel types labeled 1 through 5 on the corresponding numbered line, writing the name in red if the vessel carries arterial blood, blue if the vessel carries venous blood, and purple if the vessel carries a mixture of both.
2. Write the names of the vascular layers labeled 6 to 10 on the corresponding numbered line.
3. Color the single-layered blood vessel and the lumen of the large blood vessels pink. Color the outside layer of structures that carry arterial blood red and the outside of the structures that carry venous blood blue.
4. Draw an arrow in the box to represent the direction of blood flow.

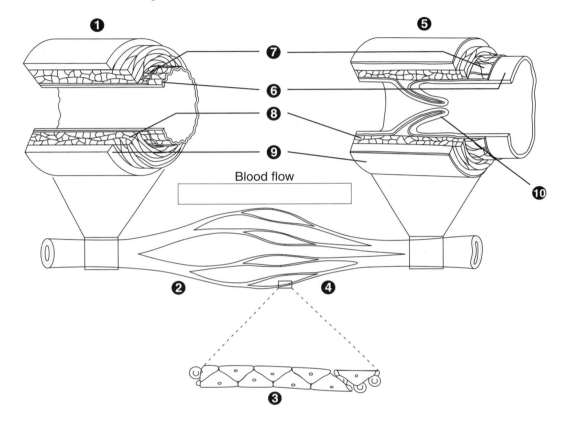

Blood flow

1. _____	6. _____
2. _____	7. _____
3. _____	8. _____
4. _____	9. _____
5. _____	10. _____

LABELING EXERCISE 6-4: REPRESENTATION OF THE VASCULAR FLOW (Text Fig. 6-10)

1. Write the name of each numbered structure or tissue on the corresponding numbered line.
2. Color deoxygenated blood flow blue and oxygenated blood flow red.
3. Draw arrows to show the direction of blood flow.

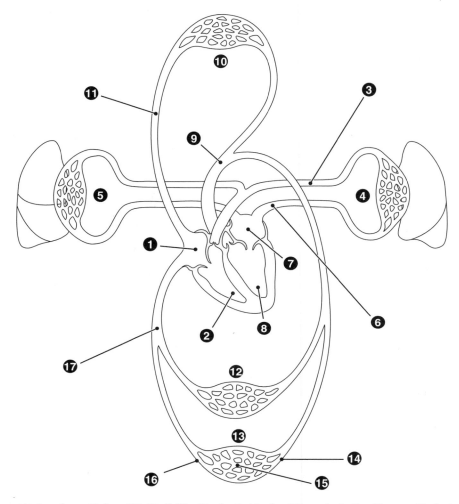

(Adapted with permission from Cohen BJ, Hull KL. *Study Guide for Memmler's the Human Body in Health and Disease,* 12th ed. Philadelphia: Lippincott Williams & Wilkins; 2013:287.)

1. _____   10. _____

2. _____   11. _____

3. _____   12. _____

4. _____   13. _____

5. _____   14. _____

6. _____   15. _____

7. _____   16. _____

8. _____   17. _____

9. _____

LABELING EXERCISE 6-5: H-SHAPED ARM VEINS (Text Fig. 6-11)

Write the name of each numbered structure on the corresponding numbered line.

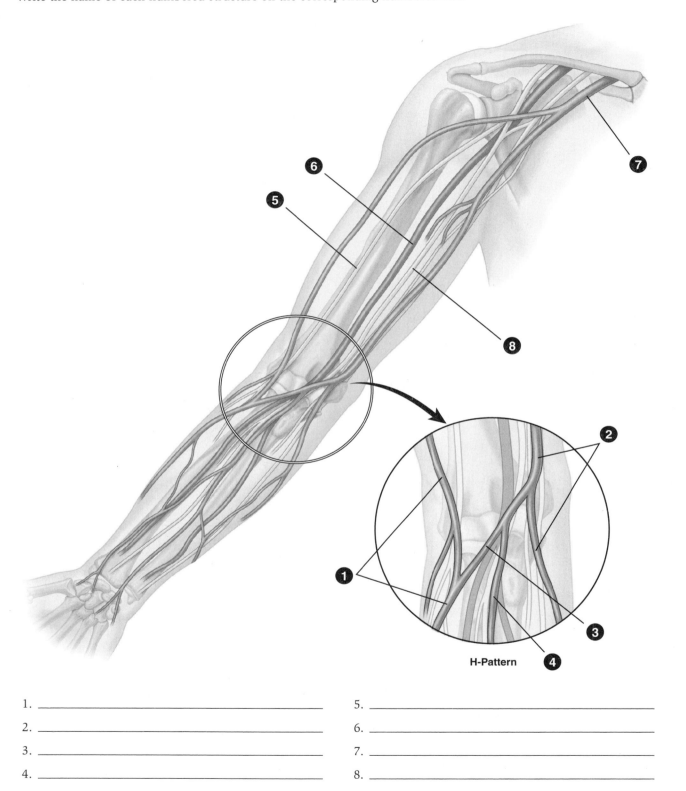

H-Pattern

1. _____

2. _____

3. _____

4. _____

5. _____

6. _____

7. _____

8. _____

LABELING EXERCISE 6-6: M-SHAPED ARM VEINS (Text Fig. 6-12)

Write the name of each numbered structure on the corresponding numbered line.

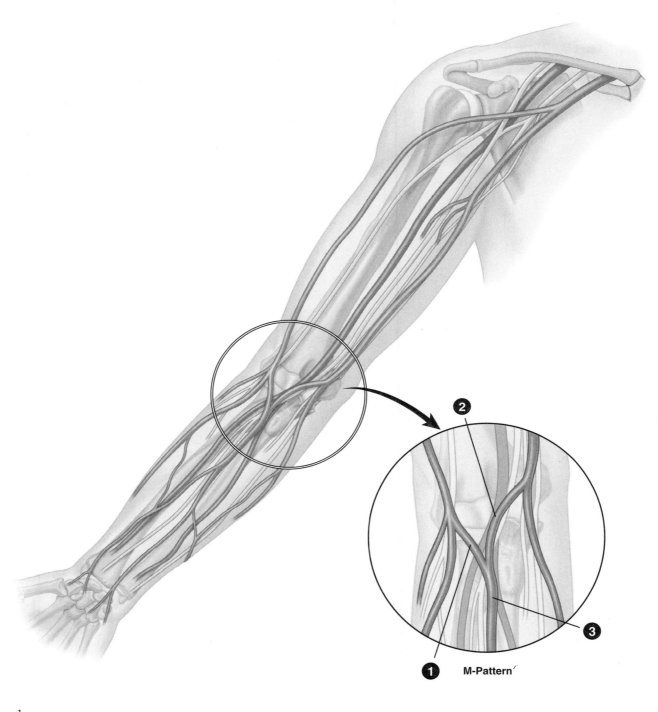

M-Pattern

1. _____

2. _____

3. _____

ABELING EXERCISE 6-7: DORSAL FOREARM, WRIST, AND HAND VEINS (Text Fig. 6-13)

Write the name of each numbered structure on the corresponding numbered line.

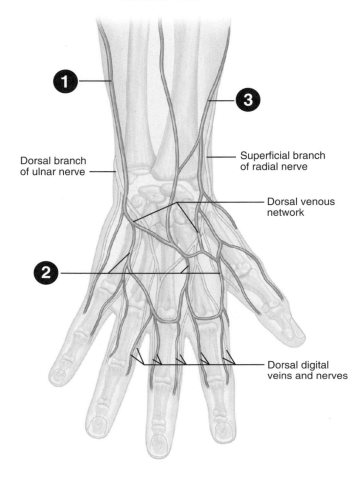

Dorsal Forearm, Wrist, and Hand Veins

Dorsal branch of ulnar nerve

Superficial branch of radial nerve

Dorsal venous network

Dorsal digital veins and nerves

1. _____

2. _____

3. _____

LABELING EXERCISE 6-8: LEG VEINS (Text Fig. 6-14)

Write the name of each numbered structure on the corresponding numbered line.

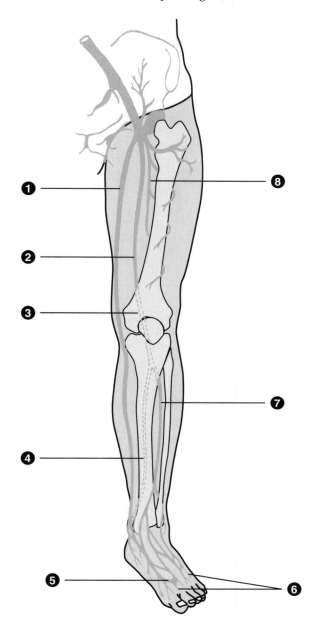

1. _____   5. _____

2. _____   6. _____

3. _____   7. _____

4. _____   8. _____

LABELING EXERCISE 6-9: WHITE BLOOD CELLS (Text Table 6-5)

1. Write the names of the types of leukocytes identified by the numbers 1 through 5 on the corresponding numbered lines.
2. Write the names of the cells or cell parts identified by numbers 6 through 9 on the corresponding numbered lines.

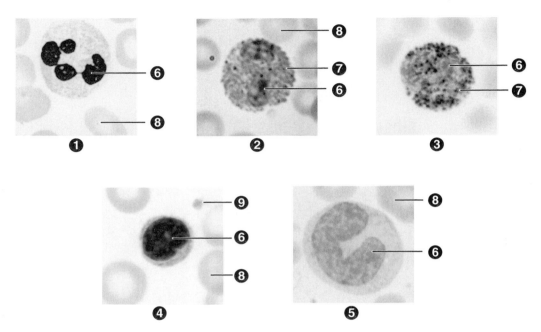

(Adapted with permission from Cohen BJ, Hull KL. *Study Guide for Memmler's the Human Body in Health and Disease,* 12th ed. Philadelphia: Lippincott Williams & Wilkins; 2013:249.)

1. _____   6. _____

2. _____   7. _____

3. _____   8. _____

4. _____   9. _____

5. _____

LABELING EXERCISE 6-10: CENTRIFUGED BLOOD SPECIMENS (Text Fig. 6-15)

1. Identify which of the following is an illustrations of a centrifuged serum specimen and which is a centrifuged whole blood specimen by writing the type of specimen on the line (A or B) next to the correct illustration.
2. Write the names of the specimen parts identified by numbers 1 through 6 on the corresponding numbered line for each specimen.

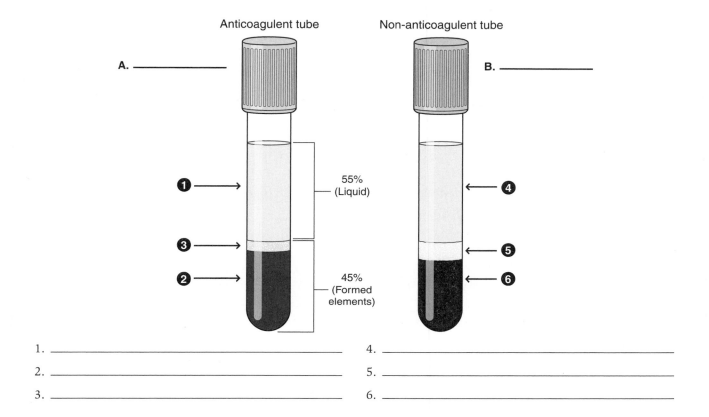

1. _____

2. _____

3. _____

4. _____

5. _____

6. _____

Knowledge Drills

KNOWLEDGE DRILL 6-1: CAUTION AND KEY POINT RECOGNITION

The following sentences have been taken from "CAUTION and KEY POINT" statements found throughout Chapter 6. Fill in the blanks with the missing information.

1. Vein (A) _____ differs somewhat from person to person and you may not see the exact TEXTBOOK pattern. The important thing to remember is to choose a (B) _____ vein that is well fixed and does not overlie a (C) _____, which indicates the presence of an (D) _____ and the potential presence of a major (E) _____.

2. The (A) _____ artery is the only artery that carries (B) _____, or oxygen-poor blood. It is part of the (C) _____ circulation and carries (D) _____ blood from the (E) _____ to the (F) _____. It is classified as an artery because it carries blood (G) _____ from the heart.

3. Natural (A) _____ circulate in the plasma along with the coagulation factors. They keep the (B) _____ process in check and limited to (C) _____ sites by (D) _____ (breaking down) any (E) _____ coagulation factors that (F) _____ the injury site or remain within the formed clot.

4. When (A) _____ blood is collected by syringe, the (B) _____ normally causes the blood to (C) _____ or _____ into the syringe under its own (D) _____.

5. Veins on the (A) _____ of the (B) _____ are never (C) _____ for venipuncture.

6. The major difference between (A) _____ and serum is: plasma contains (B)_____, while (C) _____ does not.

7. The presence of (A) _____ within (B) _____ is a major (C) _____ difference between arteries and veins.

8. Testing personnel typically prefer specimens that contain roughly (A) _____ times the amount of sample required to perform the test; so the test can be (B) _____ if needed with some to spare. Consequently, a test that requires 1 mL of (C) _____ or plasma would require a (D) _____ blood specimen because only half the specimen will be (E) _____, while a test that requires 1 mL (F) _____ blood would require a (G) _____ specimen.

9. _____ lymph nodes (nodes in the armpit) are often removed as part of (B) _____ cancer surgery. Their removal can impair (C) _____ drainage and interfere with the destruction of (D) _____ and foreign matter in the affected arm. This is cause for concern in phlebotomy and the reason an (E) _____ on the same side as a (F) _____ is not suitable for venipuncture.

10. The main component of RBCs is (A) _____ (_____ or _____), an (B) _____-containing pigment that enables them to transport (C) _____ and (D) _____ _____ and also gives them their (E) _____ _____.

KNOWLEDGE DRILL 6-2: SCRAMBLED WORDS

Unscramble the following words using the hints given in parenthesis and the letters that have been placed in the correct boxes. Finish writing the correct spelling of the scrambled words in the corresponding boxes.

1. shenioda (a platelet function)

	d	h					

2. gingatulitano (a transfusion worry)

			l			n				n

3. sidelota (part of the cardiac cycle)

		a		t			

4. philamihoe (coagulation disorder)

	e			p				

5. yomplahm (lymphatic system disorder)

	y				m	

6. pichlace (a safe vein choice)

c			h				

7. daymirmuco (the muscle behind the "pump")

				a			u	

8. nopulamrechlorpoy (describes a type of WBC)

			y			p		n							

9. nesmulria (like a half-moon)

		m					r	

10. critsovonnastico (helps prevent blood loss)

	a		o							c	t			

KNOWLEDGE DRILL 6-3: TRUE/FALSE ACTIVITY

The following statements are all false. Circle the one or two words that make the statement false and write the correct word(s) that would make the statement true in the space provided.

1. The three layers of the heart are the epicardium, the myocardium, and pericardium.

2. Cardiac contraction is initiated by an electrical impulse generated from the AV Bundle, also called the pacemaker.

3. Veins are blood vessels that carry blood away from the heart.

4. Myocardial ischemia is defined as a heart attack or death of the heart muscle due to occlusion.

5. When venous blood is collected by syringe, the pressure normally causes the blood to "pump" into the syringe.

6. Venules are microscopic, one-cell–thick vessels that connect the arteries and arterioles.

7. The venous distribution patterns are so named because the major AC veins on the arm resemble the shape of either an "H" or a "Y".

8. The AC fossa is the shallow depression in the arm that is inferior and above the bend of the elbow.

9. The "H-shaped" venous distribution pattern displayed by approximately 50% of the population includes the median cephalic vein, cephalic vein, and the basilic vein.

10. The main function of RBCs is to destroy pathogens.

11. Blood that is removed from the body will clot within 10 to 15 minutes. The blood cells are enmeshed in a fibrin network and the remaining fluid portion is called plasma.

12. Tests for lymphatic disorders include d-dimer, prothrombin time, and partial thromboplastin time.

Skills Drills

SKILLS DRILL 6-1: REQUISITION ACTIVITY

You have received the following test order. Name the circulatory system part or process associated with each test ordered. Write the answer in the margin next to the test.

Any Hospital USA
1123 West Physician Drive
Any Town USA

Laboratory Test Requisition

- -

PATIENT INFORMATION:

Name: _____ Doe _____ Jane _____ M _____
                 (last)   (first)   (MI)

Identification Number: __03265791__   Birth Date: _09/17/55_

Referring Physician: __Goodhart__

Date to be Collected: __06/22/15__   Time to be Collected: __0600__

Special Instructions: __Patient is on a blood thinner__

- -

TEST(S) REQUIRED:

_____ NH4 – Ammonia	_____ Gluc – glucose
_____ Bili – Bilirubin, total & direct	_X_ Hgb – hemoglobin
_____ BMP – basic metabolic panel	_____ Lact – lactic acid/lactate
_____ BUN - Blood urea nitrogen	_____ Plt. Ct. – platelet count
_____ Lytes – electrolytes	_X_ PT – prothrombin time
_____ CBC – complete blood count	_____ PTT – partial thromboplastin time
_X_ Chol – cholesterol	_____ RPR – rapid plasma reagin
_____ ESR – erythrocyte sed rate	_____ T&S – type and screen
_____ EtOH - alcohol	_____ PSA – prostatic specific antigen
_____ D-dime	_X_ Other __Digoxin__

SKILLS DRILL 6-2: WORD BUILDING

Divide each word into all of its elements (parts): prefix (P), word root (WR), combining vowel (CV), and suffix (S). Write the word part and its definition on the corresponding lines. Write the general meaning of the word in the space provided. If the word does not have a particular element, write NA (not applicable) in its place.

Example: Pericardium

Elements _____*peri*_____ / _____*card*_____ / _____ / _____*ium*_____
          P   WR   CV   S

Definitions _____*around*_____ / _____*heart*_____ / _____ / _____*structure*_____

Meaning: structure around the heart

1. Erythrocyte

   Elements _____ / _____ / _____ / _____
             P   WR   CV   S

   Definitions _____ / _____ / _____ / _____

   Meaning:

2. Anemia

   Elements _____ / _____ / _____ / _____
             P   WR   CV   S

   Definitions _____ / _____ / _____ / _____

   Meaning:

3. Hemostatic

   Elements _____ / _____ / _____ / _____
             P   WR   CV   S

   Definitions _____ / _____ / _____ / _____

   Meaning:

4. Endocarditis

   Elements _____ / _____ / _____ / _____
             P   WR   CV   S

   Definitions _____ / _____ / _____ / _____

   Meaning:

5. Toxic

   Elements _____ / _____ / _____ / _____
             P   WR   CV   S

   Definitions _____ / _____ / _____ / _____

   Meaning:

6. Thrombocyte

   Elements _____ / _____ / _____ / _____
             P   WR   CV   S

   Definitions _____ / _____ / _____ / _____

   Meaning:

Crossword

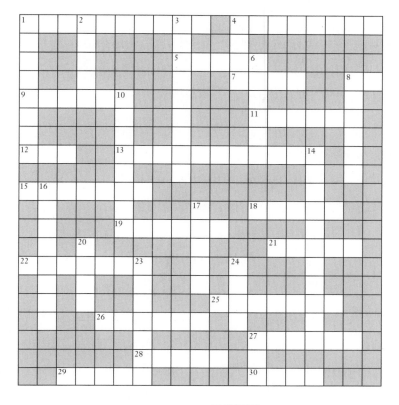

ACROSS

1. Test to determine suitability of mixing donor and recipient blood
4. Containing blood vessels
5. The upper, receiving chambers on each side of the heart
7. Lymph system structure that can remove impurities
8. Prothrombin time (abbrev.)
9. Abnormal reduction in the number of RBCs in the circulating blood
11. A coat or layer of tissue, as in a blood vessel
12. Abbreviation for a common hematology test
13. Medical term for red blood cell
15. Medication/therapy for cardiac disease
18. Fluid that circulates within the vascular system
19. Partition that separates the right and left chambers of the heart
21. Muscular organ that receives blood from veins and propels it into arteries
22. Small veins that emerge from capillaries
25. Last-choice AC vein for venipuncture
26. Another name for the bicuspid heart valve
27. Test used to identify the presence of fibrinolysis
28. Fluid derived from excess tissue fluid and similar in composition to plasma
29. Vein structure that helps keep blood flowing toward the heart
30. Soft, insoluble mass found in red-top tube

DOWN

1. Second-choice AC vein for venipuncture
2. Pale-yellow fluid that can be separated from a clotted blood specimen
3. To clot, or change from liquid to solid
4. Blood vessel that returns blood to the heart
6. Pertaining to the large artery arising from the left ventricle
8. Fluid portion of the circulating blood
10. Blood vessels that carry blood away from the heart
14. Term for the thin inner layer of the heart
16. Insufficient blood supply to an area due to obstruction of the blood vessels carrying blood to the area
17. _____ coat is composed of WBCs and platelets
20. Colloquial name for the heart, "the _____"
23. Contracting phase of the cardiac cycle
24. Immediately
27. Pathological form of diffuse coagulation (abbrev.)

Chapter Review Questions

1. The thin membrane lining the heart that is continuous with the lining of the blood vessels is the
   a. endocardium.
   b. epicardium.
   c. myocardium.
   d. pericardium.

2. Partitions that separate the right and left chambers of the heart are called
   a. chordae tendineae.
   b. cusps.
   c. Purkinje fibers.
   d. septa.

3. The bicuspid valve in the heart is also called the
   a. aortic valve.
   b. mitral valve.
   c. pulmonic valve.
   d. tricuspid valve.

4. The function of the right ventricle is to
   a. deliver blood to the aorta.
   b. deliver blood to the pulmonary artery.
   c. receive blood from the pulmonary vein.
   d. receive blood from the vena cava.

5. A fast heart rate is called
   a. arrhythmia.
   b. bradycardia.
   c. fibrillations.
   d. tachycardia.

6. The sound of the heartbeat comes from
   a. contracting myocardium.
   b. firing of the sinoatrial node.
   c. opening and closing of the valves.
   d. resonating interventricular septa.

7. Diastolic blood pressure is the pressure in the arteries during
   a. atrial contraction.
   b. atrial relaxation.
   c. ventricular contraction.
   d. ventricular relaxation.

8. Which of the following arteries carries deoxygenated blood?
   a. Brachial
   b. Femoral
   c. Pulmonary
   d. Radial

9. A vein is defined as any blood vessel that carries
   a. blood away from the heart.
   b. blood to the heart.
   c. deoxygenated blood.
   d. oxygen-rich blood.

10. While selecting a vein for venipuncture, you feel a distinct pulse. What you are feeling is a/an
    a. artery.
    b. nerve.
    c. valve.
    d. vein.

11. A major difference between veins and arteries is that
    a. arteries have a thicker external layer.
    b. arteries have no endothelial layer.
    c. veins have a thicker medial layer.
    d. veins have valves.

12. The outer layer of a blood vessel is called the tunica
    a. adventitia.
    b. interna.
    c. intima.
    d. media.

13. Which of the following veins are most commonly used for venipuncture?
    a. Basilic and median cubital
    b. Cephalic and basilic
    c. Median cubital and cephalic
    d. Radial and basilic

14. Which of the following formed elements is actually part of a bone marrow cell called a megakaryocyte?
    a. Erythrocyte
    b. Granulocyte
    c. Thrombocyte
    d. Reticulocyte

15. Whole blood consists of all of the following except
    a. cells.
    b. fibrin.
    c. plasma.
    d. solutes.

16. A person's blood type is determined by antigens on the surfaces of the
    a. eosinophils.
    b. platelets.
    c. red blood cells.
    d. white blood cells.

17. The third response of the coagulation process is
    a. fibrinolysis.
    b. platelet plug formation.
    c. hemostatic plug formation.
    d. vasoconstriction.

18. When platelets stick to each other during the coagulation process, it is called
    a. aggregation.
    b. adhesion.
    c. infarction.
    d. inhibition.

19. Which of the following is a function of the lymphatic system?
    a. Carry oxygen to the cells
    b. Regulate blood pressure
    c. Remove microorganisms
    d. Synthesize coagulation factors

20. A blood clot circulating in the bloodstream is called a/an
    a. embolism.   c. phlebitis.
    b. embolus.   d. thrombus.

21. The structure in the heart that starts the heartbeat is the
    a. AV node.   c. bundle branches.
    b. AV bundle.   d. sinoatrial node.

22. The normal ECG tracing is useful for diagnosing
    a. blood pressure abnormalities.
    b. circulatory embolism.
    c. damage to the heart muscle.
    d. pacemaker malfunction.

23. Erythrocytes main function is to
    a. carry oxygen from the lungs to the cells.
    b. engulf and destroy foreign matter.
    c. form cellular plugs to stop bleeding.
    d. release histamine and heparin.

24. A laboratory test that is ordered to evaluate the hemostatic process is
    a. bone marrow biopsy.
    b. complete blood count.
    c. prothrombin time.
    d. reticulocyte count.

Case Studies

Case Study 6-1: Circulatory System Disorders and Diagnostic Tests

A phlebotomist receives a request to collect specimens for stat electrolytes, CK, and AST on a patient with a possible MI. When the phlebotomist arrives to draw the specimen, a physician is with the patient and the patient is explaining that he had been feeling extreme anginal pains for almost an hour now. The physician tells the phlebotomist to go ahead and draw the specimen. The patient has an IV in the left arm near the wrist. There is a sphygmomanometer around the upper right arm.

QUESTIONS

1. What do the abbreviations CK and AST stand for?

2. What circulatory system structure is being evaluated by the ordered tests?

3. Tell what the abbreviation MI stands for and explain what it means in nonmedical terms.

4. What does angina have to do with the patient's possible diagnosis of MI?

5. What is a sphygmomanometer, and can the phlebotomist use that arm to draw blood?

Case Study 6-2: Circulatory System Disorders, Diagnostic Tests, and Vein Selection

A phlebotomist receives a request to collect a specimen for a PT and D-dimer on a patient. The phlebotomist remembers drawing the patient in the ER when he was complaining of leg pain. Because the patient was a difficult draw, the phlebotomist wanted to draw from an ankle vein, but the physician would not give permission. The patient was subsequently diagnosed with DVT. When the phlebotomist received the next request on this patient, he still couldn't find a good vein in the AC area, but he noticed that the patient had a large vein on the underside of the wrist. Before he could collect from the wrist area, he was called to a stat in ER.

QUESTIONS

1. Should the phlebotomist draw from the vein on the underside of the wrist? Why or why not?

2. What do PT and DVT stand for?

3. What body process is being evaluated by the requested tests?

4. What type of specimen is required: serum, plasma, or whole blood?

5. Give a reason for your selection of specimen type.

Case Study 6-3: Circulatory System Disorders, Diagnostic Tests, and Vein Selection

A phlebotomist is called to ER to draw a stat hct, hgb, and plt ct on a young girl who appears extremely pale and very close to being unconscious. While checking for a good puncture site, the phlebotomist notes the "M" pattern of veins on both arms but really can't feel the veins that well. After reapplying the tourniquet and making it a bit tighter, the vein in the middle of the AC on the right arm becomes palpable, but when entered the blood slowly drips into the tube. After the tube is filled, the phlebotomist applies pressure to the puncture site and makes a point of holding it longer than usual before applying a new gauze and tape. While waiting she overhears the nurse say that the patient's BP is 80/50 and her pulse is weak. The mother says her daughter had a nose bleed that lasted almost all night. Ready to go back to the laboratory, the phlebotomist checks the puncture site again and sees that the bleeding has not stopped. The ER tech continues to put pressure on the site as the phlebotomist leaves.

QUESTIONS

1. From which vein did the phlebotomist collect the blood specimens for the tests?

2. What do the abbreviations of the three tests that were ordered stand for?

3. What body processes or systems are being evaluated by the requested tests?

4. Why did the blood enter so slowly into the evacuated tube?

5. Why did the applied pressure and length of time not stop blood from flowing at the puncture site?

UNIT II Crossword Exercise

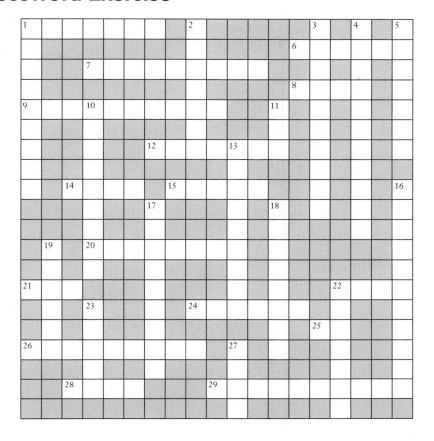

ACROSS

1. Tiny sacs in the lungs where oxygen exchange takes place
6. Fundamental working unit of the nervous system
7. Sometimes called the master gland
8. Physician's permission required for venipuncture in this area
9. Breakdown of complex substances into simple ones
12. Last-choice AC vein for venipuncture
14. A mass of lymphatic tissue through which lymph flows
15. Normally clear pale-yellow fluid that can be separated from a clotted specimen
20. Circulation pathway that carries oxygenated blood throughout the body
21. Blood group system
22. Partial thromboplastin time (pl. abbrev.)
24. Word element that precedes a word root
26. Type of gland that secretes directly into the bloodstream
28. Vessel that typically carries deoxygenated blood
29. Blood coagulation is a component of this process

DOWN

1. Without blood or lymph vessels
2. A type of cell duplication that involves doubling of DNA and cell division
3. Iron-containing pigment that gives RBCs their color
4. Medical term for red blood cell
5. The science of the structural composition of living things
10. Body process in which simple compounds are converted into complex substances
11. Widespread simultaneous clotting and fibrinolysis in the circulatory system
13. Medical term for white blood cell
16. State of equilibrium of the internal environment of the body
17. Coagulation pathway activated by tissue thromboplastin
18. Viscid fluid found in the joints
19. Protein filament formed by action of thrombin on fibrinogen
22. Coagulation cascade involves an intrinsic and extrinsic _____
23. Lying face down
27. One of the waste products of metabolism

Chapter 7

Blood Collection Equipment, Additives, and Order of Draw

Objectives

Study the information in your TEXTBOOK that corresponds to each objective to prepare yourself for the activities in this chapter.

1 List, describe, and explain the purpose of the equipment and supplies needed to collect blood specimens by venipuncture, and define associated terms and abbreviations.

2 List and describe evacuated tube system (ETS) and syringe system components, explain how each system works, and tell how to determine which system and components to use.

3 Demonstrate knowledge of the types of blood collection additives, identify the chemical composition of the specific additives within each type, and describe how each additive works.

4 Describe ETS tube stopper color coding used to identify the presence or absence of an additive, connect additives and stopper colors with laboratory departments and tests, and list the order of draw and explain its importance.

Matching

Use choices only once unless otherwise indicated.

MATCHING 7-1: KEY TERMS AND DESCRIPTIONS

Match each key term with the *best* description.

Key Terms (1–16)

1. _____ ACD
2. _____ Additive
3. _____ Anticoagulant
4. _____ Antiglycolytic agent
5. _____ Antiseptics
6. _____ Bevel
7. _____ Butterfly needle
8. _____ Clot activator
9. _____ Disinfectant
10. _____ EDTA
11. _____ ETS
12. _____ Evacuated tube
13. _____ Gauge
14. _____ Glycolysis
15. _____ Heparin
16. _____ Hub

Descriptions

A. Abbreviation for the collection system typically used for routine venipuncture
B. Additive that prevents the breakdown of glucose by the cells
C. Additive used for immunohematology tests such as DNA and HLA typing
D. Anticoagulant that inhibits the formation of thrombin
E. Anticoagulant that preserves cell shape and structure and inhibits platelet clumping
F. Breakdown or metabolism of glucose by blood cells
G. Coagulation-enhancing substance, such as silica
H. End of the needle that attaches to the blood collection device
I. Number that is related to the diameter of the needle lumen
J. Point of a needle that is cut on a slant for ease of skin entry
K. Premeasured vacuum tube that is color-coded based on its addiive
L. Solutions used to kill microorganisms on surfaces and instruments
M. Substance added to a blood collection tube
N. Substance that prevents blood from clotting
O. Substances used for skin cleaning that inhibit the growth of bacteria
P. Winged infusion blood collection set

Key Terms (17–32)

17. _____ Hypodermic needle
18. _____ Lumen
19. _____ Multisample needle
20. _____ Order of draw
21. _____ Potassium oxalate
22. _____ PST
23. _____ RST
24. _____ Shaft
25. _____ Sharps container
26. _____ Silica
27. _____ Sodium citrate
28. _____ Sodium fluoride
29. _____ SPS
30. _____ SST
31. _____ Thixotropic gel
32. _____ Winged infusion set

Descriptions

A. Additive used in blood culture collection
B. Anticoagulant commonly used to preserve coagulation factors
C. Anticoagulant commonly used with an antiglycolytic agent
D. Butterfly needle
E. Clot activator
F. Gel tube for separation of cells and serum
G. Heparinized gel tube for separation of cells and plasma
H. Internal space of a vessel or tube
I. Long cylindrical portion of a needle
J. Most common antiglycolytic agent
K. Special puncture-resistant leakproof disposable container
L. Special sequence in which tubes are filled during a multiple-tube draw
M. Synthetic substance used to separate cells from serum or plasma
N. Tube containing thrombin and gel barrier.
O. Type of needle used to collect several tubes during a single venipuncture
P. Type of needle used when collecting blood with a syringe

MATCHING 7-2: MATCH THE ADDITIVE WITH ITS PRIMARY FUNCTION

Choices may be used more than once.

Additive

1. _____ ACD

2. _____ CPD

3. _____ EDTA

4. _____ Heparin

5. _____ Potassium oxalate

6. _____ Silica

7. _____ Sodium citrate

8. _____ Sodium fluoride

9. _____ SPS

10. _____ Thixotropic gel

Primary Function

A. Anticoagulant
B. Antiglycolytic agent
C. Clot activator
D. Serum/plasma separator

MATCHING 7-3: MATCH THE ADDITIVE WITH THE TYPE OF ACTION

Choices may be used more than once.

Additive

1. _____ Citrate

2. _____ EDTA

3. _____ Heparin

4. _____ Potassium oxalate

5. _____ Silica

6. _____ Sodium fluoride

7. _____ Thixotropic gel

Type of Action

A. Binds calcium
B. Enhances coagulation
C. Inhibits thrombin
D. Physical barrier
E. Preserves glucose

Labeling Exercises

LABELING EXERCISE 7-1: TUBE STOPPER COLORS AND ADDITIVES

Color the tube stoppers of the following ETS plastic tubes according to the list of tubes below. If the tube contains gel, color the area of the tube that would contain the gel yellow. Using the list of additives, write the letter(s) of the possible tube additive(s) inside the corresponding tube. *Note:* Additive choices may be used more than once, and some tube choices may have more than one additive.

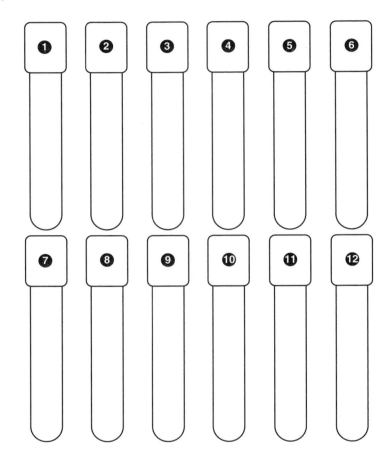

Tubes

1. Gray top
2. Green top (nongel)
3. Lavender top
4. Light-blue top
5. Pink top
6. PPT
7. PST
8. Red top
9. Royal-blue top
10. SST
11. Yellow top (blood bank)
12. Yellow top (microbiology)

Additives

A. Acid citrate dextrose (ACD)
B. Clot activator (silica)
C. EDTA
D. Heparin
E. No additive
F. Potassium oxalate
G. Sodium citrate
H. Sodium fluoride
I. Sodium polyanethol sulfonate (SPS)
J. Thixotropic gel

LABELING EXERCISE 7-2: TUBE STOPPER COLORS AND ORDER OF DRAW

Identify the stopper color of the tube required for the following types of tests assuming that they would all be collected from the same patient at the same time. Then, in the order of draw from left to right, color the stoppers of the following tubes to correspond to the tubes required for the types of tests.

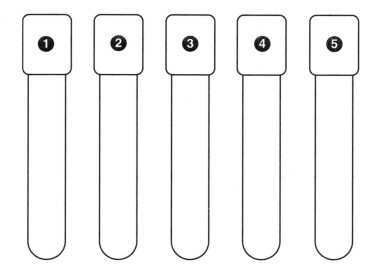

Tube Stopper Color	**Type of Test**
1. _____	Chemistry test (antiglycolytic agent required)
2. _____	Chemistry test (plasma required)
3. _____	Chemistry test (serum required)
4. _____	Coagulation test
5. _____	Hematology test

Knowledge Drills

KNOWLEDGE DRILL 7-1: CAUTION AND KEY POINT RECOGNITION

The following sentences are taken from "CAUTION AND KEY POINT" statements found throughout the text of Chapter 7. Using the TEXTBOOK, fill in the blanks with the missing information.

1. According to (A) _____ regulations, if the (B) _____ does not have a

   (C) _____ feature, the equipment it is used with (such as tube holder or syringe) must have a

   (D) _____ feature to minimize the chance of an accidental needlestick.

2. Always check the (A) _____ (B) _____ on a tube before using it, and never use a tube

   that has (C) _____ or has been (D) _____.

3. An underfilled (A) _____ tube will have an incorrect blood-to-additive (B) _____, which

   can cause (C) _____ test results.

4. Cleaning with an (A) _____ reduces the number of (B) _____ but does not

   (C) _____ the site.

5. (A) _____ of hands after (B) _____ removal is essential.

6. Heparinized (A) _____ is preferred over (B) _____ for (C) _____ tests

   because when blood clots, (D) _____ is released from (E) _____ into the serum

   and can falsely elevate results.

7. If (A) _____ are detected in a (B) _____ specimen, it cannot be used for

   testing and must be (C) _____.

8. *Never* (A) _____ or otherwise (B) _____ (C) _____ a specimen, as

   this can cause (D) _____, which makes most specimens unsuitable for testing.

9. *Never* transfer blood collected in an (A) _____ tube into another (B) _____

   tube, even if the (C) _____ are the same.

10. (A) _____ regulations require that the tube holder with (B) _____ (C) _____

    be disposed of as a (D) _____ after use and never be removed from the (E) _____ and

    reused.

11. The (A) _____ tube collected with a (B) _____ will underfill because of

    (C) _____ in the tubing. If the tube contains an (D) _____, the blood-to-additive ratio

    will be affected.

12. The (A) _____ ratio of blood to (B) _____ in light-blue (C) _____

    (D) _____ tubes is (E) _____; therefore, it is extremely important to fill them to the

    stated volume.

KNOWLEDGE DRILL 7-2: SCRAMBLED WORDS

Unscramble the following words using the hints given in parenthesis and the letters that have been placed in the correct boxes. Finish writing the correct spelling of the scrambled word in the corresponding boxes.

1. cavmuu (negative pressure)

	a			u	

2. clabeh (sodium hypochlorite)

			a	c	

3. eggua (measure of diameter)

			g	

4. mulen (the space within)

		m		

5. pheanri (it inhibits thrombin)

				r	i	

6. poxihirctot (type of gel)

		i				o		i	

7. quinretout (used to restrict blood flow)

		u		n			e	

8. reatict (coagulation tube additive)

				a	t	

9. treyfblut (winged infusion set)

			t	e			y	

10. veldrean (EDTA tube stopper color)

			e		e	

11. voyarcrer (transfer from one tube to another)

		r	y		e	

12. zitsieran (used to decontaminate hands)

			i		i		e	

KNOWLEDGE DRILL 7-3: TRUE/FALSE ACTIVITY

The following statements are all false. Circle the one or two words that make the statement false and write the correct word/s that would make the statement true in the space provided.

1. Use of bandaids to hold pressure is not recommended because they tend to stick to the site and reinitiate bleeding when removed because they dislodge the platelet plug that seals a puncture site.

2. A properly applied tourniquet is tight enough to restrict arterial flow out of the area but not so tight as to restrict venous flow into the area.

3. A needle or tube holder that has a safety device is an example of a SESIP, which is the CLIA acronym for a sharp with engineered sharps injury protection.

4. When drawing venous blood by syringe, the phlebotomist slowly pulls back the plunger, creating a vacuum that causes the shaft to fill with blood.

5. A transfer device must be held horizontal when tubes are being filled in order to prevent blood in the tube from touching the needle in the transfer device.

6. An additive tube must be gently inverted two to four times, depending on the type of additive and the manufacturer, immediately after collection to adequately mix the additive with the specimen.

7. Vigorous mixing or an excessive number of inversions in light blue tubes can activate white cells and lengthen clotting times.

8. When using the ETS system, royal-blue tops for trace element studies should be collected first to avoid even the smallest amount of carryover.

9. The most common antimicrobial agent is **sodium fluoride.** It preserves glucose and also inhibits the growth of bacteria.

10. Sodium fluoride in tubes has been the source of more carryover problems than any other additive.

KNOWLEDGE DRILL 7-4: STOPPER COLORS, ADDITIVES, AND DEPARTMENTS

Fill in the blanks of the following table with the missing information.

Stopper Color(s)	Additive	Department(s)
Light blue	Sodium citrate	(1) _____
Red (glass)	(2) _____	Chemistry, Blood Bank, Serology/Immunology
Red (plastic)	Clot activator	(3) _____
Red/light gray	(4) _____	NA (discard purpose only)
Clear		
Red/black (tiger)	Clot activator and	Chemistry
(5) _____	(6) _____	
Green/gray	Lithium heparin and gel separator	Chemistry
(7) _____		
Green	Lithium heparin	(8) _____
	Sodium heparin	
Lavender (purple)	EDTA	(9) _____
(10) _____	EDTA	Blood Bank
Gray	Sodium fluoride and	Chemistry
	(11) _____	
	Sodium fluoride and	
	(12) _____	
	Sodium fluoride	
Orange	(13) _____	Chemistry
Gray/yellow		
Royal blue	(14) _____	Chemistry
	(15) _____	
	Sodium (16) _____	
Tan (plastic)	(17) _____	Chemistry
Yellow	(18) _____ _____ (SPS)	Microbiology
Yellow	Acid citrate dextrose (19) (_____)	(20) _____ / Immunohematology

Skills Drills

SKILLS DRILL 7-1: REQUISITION ACTIVITY

Identify the tests ordered on the following requisition. List the tests below in the order of draw and identify the stopper color and additive of the tubes that will most likely be collected for the tests indicated.

Test in Order of Draw   **Tube Stopper Color and Additive**

1. _____   _____

2. _____   _____

3. _____   _____

4. _____   _____

Any Hospital USA
1123 West Physician Drive
Any Town USA

Laboratory Test Requisition

PATIENT INFORMATION:

Name: _____ Doe _____ John _____ T _____
                (last)   (first)   (MI)
Identification Number: __036152912__   Birth Date: 12/07/43

Referring Physician: __Smarte, John__

Date to be Collected: __06/28/2015__   Time to be Collected: _____

Special Instructions: __**STAT**__

TEST(S) ORDERED:

Chemistry		Coagulation	
	NH4 (Ammonia)		D-dimer
	Bili (Bilirubin, total & direct)	√	PT (protime)
	BMP (basic metabolic panel)		PTT (partial thromboplastin time)
	BUN (Blood urea nitrogen)	**Hematology**	
	Chol (cholesterol)		CBC (complete blood count)
	EtOH (alcohol)		ESR (erythrocyte sed rate)
	Gluc (glucose)		Hgb (hemoglobin)
√	Lytes (electrolytes)	√	H & H (hemoglobin & Hematocrit)
	Lact (lactic acid/lactate)		RBC (Red blood cell count)
	PSA (prostatic specific antigen)		WBC (White blood cell count)
Other	√	Type & Screen (serum specimen requested)	

SKILLS DRILL 7-2: WORD BUILDING

Divide each word into all of its elements (parts); prefix (P), word root (WR), combining vowel (CV), and suffix (S). Write the word part and its definition on the corresponding lines. Write the general meaning of the word in the space provided. If the word does not have a particular element, write NA (not applicable) in its place.

Example: Antiglycolytic

Elements _____*anti*_____ / _____*glyc*_____ / _____*o*_____ / _____*lytic*_____
                    P   WR   CV   S

Definitions _____*against*_____ / _____*sugar*_____ / _____*NA*_____ / _*pertaining to breakdown*_

Meaning: Against the breakdown of sugar (glucose)

1. Hypodermic

   Elements _____ / _____ / _____ / _____
                       P   WR   CV   S

   Definitions _____ / _____ / _____ / _____

   Meaning:

2. Dermatitis

   Elements _____ / _____ / _____ / _____
                       P   WR   CV   S

   Definitions _____ / _____ / _____ / _____

   Meaning:

3. Antiseptic

   Elements _____ / _____ / _____ / _____
                       P   WR   CV   S

   Definitions _____ / _____ / _____ / _____

   Meaning:

4. Microorganism

   Elements _____ / _____ / _____ / _____
                       P   WR   CV   S

   Definitions _____ / _____ / _____ / _____

   Meaning:

5. Vascular

   Elements _____ / _____ / _____ / _____
                       P   WR   CV   S

   Definitions _____ / _____ / _____ / _____

   Meaning:

6. Intradermal

   Elements _____ / _____ / _____ / _____
                       P   WR   CV   S

   Definitions _____ / _____ / _____ / _____

   Meaning:

Crossword

ACROSS

2. EDTA or oxalate anticoagulants are usually salts of this element
5. Diameter of the lumen of the needle
8. Winged infusion set
10. Solution used to remove or kill microbes
12. It forms in a tube of blood that does not have anticoagulant in it
16. Used to clean the site before puncture (plural)
17. Another name for cap on evacuated tubes
18. Internal space of a tube or blood vessel
19. Used to obtain blood when veins are very fragile
21. Gold-top tube that contains separator gel (abbrev.)
22. Any substance added to an evacuated collection tube
23. Agency that mandates and enforces safe working conditions
25. The time it takes to turn around test results
29. End of the needle that is cut on a slant for ease of insertion
31. Inflammation of the skin
32. Type of examination glove
33. Only clot activator is found in this plastic evacuated tube
34. Phlebotomy standards are set by this institute

DOWN

1. Name for a sterile syringe needle
2. Heparin gel-barrier tube (abbrev.)
3. Clot activator in SST
4. Short for microorganisms
6. Literally means "against glucose breakdown"
7. Type of needle used with an ETS
9. Barrier used in separator tubes, thixotropic _____
11. Items needed for phlebotomy procedure
13. Tiny clots invisible to the eye
14. 21-gauge or 22-gauge _____
15. EDTA gel barrier tube (abbrev.)
20. ETS cap color that indicates EDTA
21. This device must be activated before a needle is discarded
24. ETS part that contains the tube during venipuncture (plural)
26. Agency that regulates food and drugs (abbrev.)
27. Name of a vessel that returns blood to the heart
28. Object on which a blood smear is made
30. Tube used to collect blood alcohol

Chapter Review Questions

1. An antiglycolytic agent
   a. enhances coagulation.
   b. inhibits thrombin formation.
   c. keeps the specimen from clotting.
   d. prevents the breakdown of glucose.

2. Sharps containers do not have to be
   a. marked "biohazard."
   b. disposable.
   c. puncture resistant.
   d. recyclable.

3. Which of the following substances would be the best thing to use to disinfect a blood spill on a lab countertop prior to cleanup?
   a. A 1:10 dilution of bleach
   b. 70% isopropyl alcohol
   c. Antibacterial soap and water
   d. Povidone–iodine swab sticks

4. This needle is the standard needle for routine venipuncture.
   a. 20 gauge   c. 22 gauge
   b. 21 gauge   d. 23 gauge

5. Needles are color coded according to
   a. expiration date.   c. length.
   b. gauge.   d. manufacturer.

6. The most common, direct, and efficient means of venipuncture is
   a. butterfly and tube holder.
   b. butterfly and syringe.
   c. ETS needle and tube holder.
   d. needle and syringe.

7. Which of the following would be the best choice of equipment for drawing a small hand vein?
   a. A 21-gauge needle and syringe
   b. A 22-gauge needle and ETS holder
   c. A 23-gauge butterfly and ETS holder
   d. A 25-gauge butterfly needle and syringe

8. Which of the following equipment is required when collecting blood by syringe?
   a. Multisample needle
   b. Tube holder
   c. Transfer device
   d. Winged infusion set

9. Which anticoagulant prevents coagulation by inhibiting thrombin formation?
   a. EDTA   c. Sodium citrate
   b. Heparin   d. Potassium oxalate

10. Which of the following tubes would typically be used to collect plasma for a stat chemistry specimen?
    a. Light-blue top   c. Red top
    b. Green top   d. Yellow top

11. EDTA is a(n)
    a. anticoagulant.
    b. clot activator.
    c. glucose preservative.
    d. plasma separator.

12. A light-blue–topped tube is most often associated with tests in this department.
    a. Chemistry   c. Hematology
    b. Coagulation   d. Serology

13. Of the following tubes, which would be filled second from a syringe according to the CLSI recommended order of draw?
    a. Gray top   c. Light-blue top
    b. Lavender top   d. Green top

14. A PST contains
    a. citrate and gel.   c. heparin and gel.
    b. EDTA and gel.   d. silica and gel.

15. Of the following tubes or containers which is filled first in the ETS order of draw?
    a. Lavender top   c. PST
    b. Light-blue top   d. SPS

16. For which of the following tubes is the blood-to-additive ratio most critical?
    a. Green top   c. Light-blue top
    b. Lavender top   d. Red top

17. Which of the following additives provides a physical barrier to prevent glycolysis?
    a. EDTA   c. Sodium fluoride
    b. Silica   d. Thixotropic gel

18. Which of the following tubes contains an anticoagulant that works by binding calcium?
    a. Green top   c. PST
    b. Light-blue top   d. SST

19. What is the purpose of a royal-blue–topped tube?
    a. Minimize trace element contamination
    b. Prevent the breakdown of glucose
    c. Prevent the specimen from clotting
    d. Protect the specimen from light

20. It is not recommended that this type of glove be worn in healthcare settings.
    a. Latex
    b. Nitrile
    c. Neoprene
    d. Vinyl

Case Studies

Case Study 7-1: Butterfly Use and Order of Draw

Maria, who was recently hired in her first job as a phlebotomist, has been sent to the ICU to collect a stat hemoglobin and hematocrit (H&H) and protime on a patient. The patient is an elderly woman whose left arm has an intravenous (IV) line. Maria checks the right arm and finds a small but suitable vein. She decides to use a butterfly with the evacuated tube system and selects the following tubes from her blood collection equipment carrier: a light-blue top for the protime, which is a coagulation test, and a lavender top for the H&H, which is a hematology test. The patient's nurse asks Maria how long she thinks it will take because she wants to give the patient a shot in that arm. Maria tells her that she has only two tubes to collect, so it shouldn't take long. The nurse leaves. Maria makes a successful venipuncture, fills the light-blue–topped tube and mixes it gently by inverting it four times. Then she fills the lavender-top tube. After finishing the draw, properly labeling the tubes, and checking and bandaging her patient, she returns to the lab. Specimen processing immediately rejects the protime and asks her to recollect it.

QUESTIONS

1. Why do you think specimen processing rejected the protime?

2. How did the way Maria collected the specimen cause the problem?

3. Why does the lab reject tubes with this problem?

4. What can Maria do differently when she recollects the specimen?

Case Study 7-2: Syringe Use and Order of Draw

A phlebotomist named Jeff has a request to collect a CBC on a postop patient. He has drawn the patient before and is aware that the patient is a "difficult" draw. He elects to use a 5-mL syringe and a 22-gauge needle on a small cephalic vein on the patient's right arm. The venipuncture is successful, and Jeff is in the middle of filling the syringe when the patient's nurse enters the room and tells him that the patient's physician wants to add electrolytes to the request. Jeff tells her that it is not a problem; he will collect a green-top tube also. He finishes the draw, attaches a transfer device, and quickly grabs the smallest tubes he can find, a 3-mL green top for the electrolytes and a 3-mL lavender top for the CBC. He puts 2 mL of blood into the green top and then 3 mL into the lavender top. He labels the tubes and writes "difficult draw" on the green top. Later a chemistry technician tells him that the patient's sodium results are off the wall and contamination is suspected. He is asked to redraw the specimen.

QUESTIONS

1. Could the problem have to do with the order of draw? Why or why not?

2. What else could have caused the problem?

3. Technically, there is another problem with the green top Jeff collected. What is it?

Case Study 7-3: A Difficult Draw

Vicki is part of the phlebotomy team in a major hospital. Today people on 04:30 shift called in sick, so the team is behind in completing the morning draws. When Vicki finally reaches her last patient she is tired, her feet hurt, and she just wants to get finished and take a break. The tests ordered are a CBC and electrolytes. Vicki cannot find a suitable antecubital vein to draw, so she decides to use a hand vein. She selects an SST and a lavender top for the draw. Blood fills the SST slowly. She is afraid the blood will stop coming, so she removes it when it is about half full, puts it in her tube holder, and engages the lavender top. The lavender is barely ¼ full when the blood stops flowing and she cannot get it going again, so she discontinues the draw. She gives the lavender-top tube a couple of quick shakes and then picks up the SST to mix it, but it has already clotted. Upon returning to the lab, she submits both specimens for processing, telling the processor it was a difficult draw and heads off on her break. The processor rejects the lavender top but accepts the SST for testing.

QUESTIONS

1. Which tube was for the CBC and which one was for the electrolytes?

2. What is the additive in each of the tubes?

3. Vicki handled both specimens incorrectly. What did she do wrong and what result could the incorrect handling have on the specimen, the testing process or test results?

4. Why would specimen processing accept the partially filled SST tube, but not the lavender top?

Chapter 8

Venipuncture Procedures

Objectives

Study the information in your TEXTBOOK that corresponds to each objective to prepare yourself for the activities in this chapter.

1 Demonstrate knowledge of each venipuncture step from the time the test request is received until the specimen is delivered to the lab, and define associated terminology.

2 Describe how to perform a venipuncture using ETS, syringe, or butterfly, list required patient and specimen identification information, describe how to handle patient ID discrepancies, and state the acceptable reasons for inability to collect a specimen.

3 Identify challenges and unique aspects associated with collecting specimens from pediatric and geriatric patients.

4 Describe why a patient would require dialysis and how it is performed, and exhibit an awareness of the type of care provided for long-term care, home care, and hospice patients.

Matching

Use each choice only once unless otherwise indicated.

MATCHING 8-1: KEY TERMS AND DESCRIPTIONS

Match each key term with the *best* description.

Key Terms (1–12)

1. _____ Accession

2. _____ Anchor

3. _____ Arm/wrist band

4. _____ ASAP

5. _____ Barcode

6. _____ Bedside manner

7. _____ Belonephobia

8. _____ DNR/DNAR

9. _____ EMLA

10. _____ Fasting

11. _____ Hospice

12. _____ ID band/bracelet

Descriptions

A. A eutectic mixture of local anesthetics

B. As soon as possible

C. Behavior of a healthcare provider toward a patient or as perceived by a patient

D. Do not resuscitate/do not attempt resuscitation

E. Identification bracelet (abbrev.)

F. No food or drink except water for 8 to 12 hours

G. Record in the order received

H. Secure firmly, as in holding a vein in place by pulling the skin taut with the thumb

I. Series of black stripes and white spaces that correspond to letters and numbers

J. The persistent, irrational fear of needles

K. Type of care for terminally ill patients

L. Two other names for an identification band/bracelet

Key Terms (13–24)

13. _____ ID card

14. _____ MR number

15. _____ Needle phobia

16. _____ Needle sheath

17. _____ NPO

18. _____ Palpate

19. _____ Patency

20. _____ Patient ID

21. _____ Preop/postop

22. _____ Reflux

23. _____ Requisition

24. _____ Stat

Descriptions

A. Backflow of blood from the tube into the vein during a draw

B. Before an operation or surgery/after an operation or surgery

C. Clinic-issued patient identification document

D. Covering or cap of a needle

E. Form on which test orders are entered and sent to the lab

F. Immediately (from the Latin *statim*, meaning "immediately")

G. Intense fear of needles

H. Medical record number used for patient ID

I. Nothing by mouth (from Latin *nil per os*)

J. Process of verifying a patient's identity

K. State of being freely open

L. To examine by feel or touch

MATCHING 8-2: SITUATION AND ACTION

Match the following venipuncture procedure situations with an acceptable action to take.

Situation

1. _____ Conflicting permission statement

2. _____ ID band not on the patient's arm

3. _____ Needle-phobic patient

4. _____ Outpatient is chewing gum

5. _____ Patient asks for the purpose of the test

6. _____ Patient initially objects to testing

7. _____ Specimen must be fasting but patient has eaten

8. _____ Unconscious patient

9. _____ You are a phlebotomy student

10. _____ You need to verify patient ID

Action

A. Actively involve the patient in this procedure.

B. Advise the patient to ask the nurse or physician.

C. Ask someone to help steady the patient's arm.

D. Ask the patient to remove it.

E. Check the ankle after asking the patient's permission.

F. Consult with the nurse or physician before proceeding.

G. Do not draw blood without the patient's consent.

H. Have the most skilled phlebotomist draw the specimen.

I. Make certain that the patient knows this information.

J. Remind the patient that the doctor needs the test results.

MATCHING 8-3: GERIATRIC PATIENT TESTS AND INDICATIONS FOR ORDERING

Match the test commonly ordered on geriatric patients (Text Table 8-3) to the typical indication for ordering.

Test

1. _____ ANA/RNA/RF

2. _____ CBC

3. _____ BUN/creatinine

4. _____ Calcium/magnesium

5. _____ Electrolytes

6. _____ ESR

7. _____ Glucose

8. _____ PT/PTT

9. _____ SPEP, IPEP

10. _____ VDRL/FTA

Typical Indication for Ordering

A. Detect and monitor diabetes. Abnormal levels can cause confusion, seizures, or coma or lead to peripheral neuropathy.

B. Detect inflammation; identify collagen vascular (i.e., connective tissue) diseases.

C. Determine hemoglobin levels, detect infection, and identify blood disorders.

D. Determine sodium and potassium levels critical to proper nervous system function.

E. Diagnose kidney function disorders that may be responsible for problems such as confusion, coma, seizures, and tremors.

F. Diagnose lupus and rheumatoid arthritis, which can affect nervous system function.

G. Identify abnormal levels associated with seizures and muscle problems.

H. Identify protein or immune globulin disorders that can lead to nerve damage.

I. Monitor blood-thinning medications; important in heart conditions, coagulation problems, and stroke management.

J. Diagnose or rule out syphilis, which can cause nerve damage and dementia.

Labeling Exercises

LABELING EXERCISE 8-1: PATIENT ID AND BLOOD SPECIMEN LABEL

You correctly identified and collected a CBC specimen on May 03, 2015, at 08:15 hours from an inpatient who was wearing the ID band shown below. Fill out the label for this patient's specimen on the tube shown below. Color the tube stopper the correct color for the test that was collected.

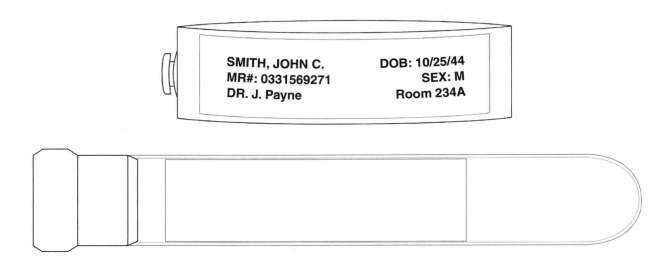

SMITH, JOHN C.   DOB: 10/25/44
MR#: 0331569271   SEX: M
DR. J. Payne   Room 234A

LABELING EXERCISE 8-2: REQUISITION AND BLOOD SPECIMEN LABEL

You correctly identified and collected a blood specimen from an inpatient at 06:00 hours using the following requisition. Fill out the label for this specimen on the tube shown below. Color the tube stopper the correct color for the test that was collected.

Any Hospital USA
1123 West Physician Drive
Any Town USA

Laboratory Test Requisition

- -

PATIENT INFORMATION:

Name: _____ Doe _____ Jane _____ A _____
           (last)   (first)   (MI)
Identification Number: __0331724395__   Birth Date: __06/14/65__

Referring Physician: __Coleman__

Date to be Collected: __05/04/2015__   Time to be Collected: __0600__

Special Instructions: __NA__

- -

TEST(S) REQUIRED:

_____ NH4 – Ammonia	_____ Gluc – glucose
_____ Bili – Bilirubin, total & direct	_____ Hgb – hemoglobin
_____ BMP – basic metabolic panel	_____ Lact – lactic acid/lactate
_____ BUN – Blood urea nitrogen	_____ Plt. Ct. – platelet count
_____ Lytes – electrolytes	__X__ PT – prothrombin time
_____ CBC – complete blood count	_____ PTT – partial thromboplastin time
_____ Chol – cholesterol	_____ RPR – rapid plasma reagin
_____ ESR – erythrocyte sed rate	_____ T&S – type and screen
_____ EtOH – alcohol	_____ PSA – prostate specific antigen
_____ D-dimer	Other _____

Knowledge Drills

KNOWLEDGE DRILL 8-1: CAUTION AND KEY POINT RECOGNITION

The following sentences are taken from "CAUTION and KEY POINT" statements found throughout Chapter 8 TEXTBOOK. Using the TEXTBOOK, fill in the blanks with the missing information.

1. *Never* verify information from an ID band that is not (A) _____ to the (B) _____, or collect a (C) _____ from an inpatient who is not (D) _____ an ID band.

2. *Never* collect a (A) _____ without some way to positively (B) _____ that specimen to the (C) _____.

3. *Do not* use veins on the (A) _____ of the wrist because (B) _____ lie close to the (C) _____ in this area and can be easily injured.

4. Remember, a patient has the (A) _____ to (B) _____ testing.

5. For safety reasons, *do not* use a two-(A) _____ technique (also called the (B) _____ hold) in which the entry point of the vein is (C) _____ by the (D) _____ finger above and the (E) _____ below.

6. If the (A) _____ end of the tube fills first, blood in the tube is in contact with the (B) _____ and (C) _____ can occur if there is a change in (D) _____ in the patient's vein.

7. Laboratory personnel will assume that blood in (A) _____ is capillary blood. If (B) _____ blood is placed in a (C) _____, it is important to label the specimen as (D) _____ blood because reference ranges for some tests differ depending on the (E) _____ of the specimen.

8. When identifying a patient *never* say, for example, (A) "_____ (B) _____ Mrs. Smith?" A person who is very (C) _____, hard of hearing, or (D) _____ may say (E) "_____" to anything.

9. A phlebotomist must be able to recognize a (A) _____ to avoid damaging it as it is the (B) _____ patient's (C) _____.

10. *Never* attempt to collect a blood specimen from a (A) _____ patient. Such an attempt may (B) _____ the patient and cause (C) _____ to the patient or the phlebotomist.

11. Never use force to (A) _____ a patient's arm or open a (B) _____, as it can cause pain and (C) _____.

12. An (A) _____ patient may be able to feel (B) _____ and (C) _____ when you (D) _____ the needle, so it may be necessary to have someone assist you in holding the arm during the blood draw.

13. A common (A) _____ and one that is irritating to the (B) _____ impaired is to (C) _____ your voice when you are speaking to them.

14. (A) _____ births present an increased risk of (B) _____ error.

15. (A) _____ a crying child as soon as possible, because the (B) _____ of crying and struggling can (C) _____ blood components and lead to (D) _____ test results.

KNOWLEDGE DRILL 8-2: SCRAMBLED WORDS

Unscramble the following words using the hints given in parenthesis and the letters that have been placed in the correct boxes. Finish writing the correct spelling of the scrambled word in the corresponding box.

1. pleonobbahie (describes a type of fear)

				n	e					i	

2. cutecite (easily melted)

	u		e				

3. cyanept (required of a vein before a draw)

				n		

4. darictipe (pertaining to children)

			i			r		

5. gnistaf (testing requirement)

					n	

6. hipabo (intense fear)

				i	

7. leaptap (a way to examine a vein)

			p			

8. narcho (firmly secure)

		c			

9. pheosic (terminal care)

			p			

10. scenicaso (record in order)

		c				o	

11. striniequio (required order)

					s			i		

12. triecagri (aged)

				a	t			

KNOWLEDGE DRILL 8-3: TRUE/FALSE ACTIVITY

The following statements are all false. Circle the one or two words that make the statement false and write the correct word/s that would make the statement true in the space provided.

1. When a computer-generated label is used, the phlebotomist is typically required to write the time of receipt and the date of collection.

2. To avoid ID and mislabeling errors, inpatient facilities require what is referred to as 2-Way ID.

3. Do not use veins on the top side of the wrist because nerves lie close to the veins in that area.

4. Either the needle, tube holder, or syringe selected must have a CLSI-required safety feature to help protect the user from accidental needlesticks.

5. After establishing the blood flow, release the tourniquet and ask the patient to squeeze the fist.

6. Although butterflies are available in various gauges, a 25-gauge butterfly is most commonly used for small and difficult veins.

7. For an antecubital site venipuncture, insert the needle into the skin at an angle of 30 degrees or more, depending on the depth of the vein.

8. The Joint Commission recommends that procedures be in place to monitor the amount of blood that is drawn from pediatric, geriatric, and other vulnerable patients to avoid phlebotomy-induced anemia.

9. Laboratory testing personnel will assume that blood in microtubes is venous blood.

10. Venipuncture in children under the age of 2 should be limited to hand veins and not deep and hard-to-find veins.

KNOWLEDGE DRILL 8-4: COMMON TEST STATUS DESIGNATIONS (Text Table 8-1)

Fill in the blanks with the missing information.

Status	Meaning	When Used	Collection Conditions	Test Examples	Priority
(1) _____	Immediately (from Latin *statim*)	Test results are urgently needed on critical patients.	Immediately collect, test, and report results. Alert lab staff when (2) _____. ER stats typically have priority over other stats.	Glucose (3) _____ Electrolytes Cardiac enzymes	First
Med Emerg	Medical Emergency (replaces stat)	Same as stat	Same as stat	Same as stat	(4) _____
Timed	Collect at a specific time	Tests for which timing is critical for accurate (5) _____	Collect as close as possible to requested time. (6) _____ actual time collected	2-hour PP (7) _____ Cortisol Cardiac enzymes (8) _____ Blood cultures	Second

(9) _____	As soon as possible	Test results are needed soon to respond to a (10) _____ situation, but patient is not critical.	Follow hospital protocol for type of test	Electrolytes Glucose H&H	(11) _____ or third depending on test
Fasting	No (12) _____ or drink except water for 8–12 hr prior to specimen collection	To eliminate diet effects on test results.	Verify that patient has fasted. If patient has not fasted, check to see if specimen should still be collected.	(13) _____ Cholesterol Triglycerides	(14) _____
NPO	Nothing by (15) _____ (From Latin *nil per os*)	Prior to surgery or other anesthesia procedures.	Do not give patient food or (16) _____ Refer requests to physician or nurse.	N/A	N/A
(17) _____	Before an operation	To determine patient eligibility for (18) _____.	Collect before the patient goes to surgery.	CBC, PTT, Platelet function studies	Same as (19) _____
Postop	After an operation	To assess patient condition after surgery.	Collect when patient is out of surgery.	(20) _____	Same as (21) _____
(22) _____	Relating to established procedure	Used to establish a diagnosis or monitor a patient's progress.	Collect in a timely manner but no urgency involved. Typically collected on morning sweeps or the next scheduled sweep.	CBC (23) _____ _____	(24) _____

KNOWLEDGE DRILL 8-5: TOURNIQUET RATIONALE

Answer the following questions in the space provided.

1. What does a tourniquet do and why is it needed in venipuncture procedures?

_____

_____

_____

2. Why is a tourniquet placed 3 to 4 inches above the intended venipuncture site?

_____

_____

_____

3. Where is the tourniquet placed in drawing blood from a hand vein?

_____

_____

_____

4. What happens if too much tension is applied in fastening a tourniquet?

_____

_____

_____

5. What is the purpose of the loop created during tourniquet application?

_____

_____

_____

6. Why is it important to release the tourniquet within 1 minute of application?

_____

_____

_____

KNOWLEDGE DRILL 8-6: GERIATRIC CHALLENGES

The text lists five challenges associated with collecting specimens from geriatric patients. One is "Effects of disease." Identify the four other challenges, describe how each can affect the specimen collection process, and explain how you would handle each one.

1. Challenge: _____

   Effect: _____

   _____

   _____

How to handle: _____

_____

_____

_____

_____

2. Challenge: _____

   Effect: _____

_____

_____

   How to handle: _____

_____

_____

_____

3. Challenge: _____

   Effect: _____

_____

_____

_____

   How to handle: _____

_____

_____

_____

_____

4. Challenge: _____

   Effect: _____

_____

_____

   How to handle: _____

_____

_____

Skills Drills

SKILLS DRILL 8-1: REQUISITION ACTIVITY (Text Fig. 8-2)

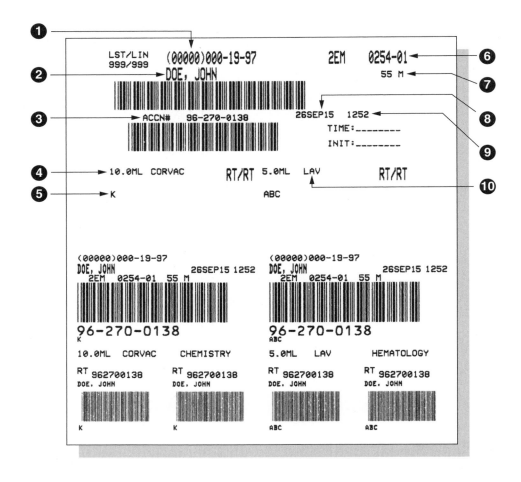

Identify each numbered item on the requisition and write the answer on the corresponding line below.

1. _____ 6. _____

2. _____ 7. _____

3. _____ 8. _____

4. _____ 9. _____

5. _____ 10. _____

SKILLS DRILL 8-2: WORD BUILDING

Divide each word into all of its elements; prefix (P), word root (WR), combining vowel (CV), and suffix (S). Write the word part and its definition on the corresponding lines. Write the general meaning of the word in the space provided. If the word does not have a particular word part, write NA (not applicable) in its place.

Example: Geriatric

Elements _____*gers*_____ / _____*iatr*_____ / _____*ic*_____
                  P   WR   S

Definitions _____*seniors*_____ / _____*treatment*_____ / _____NA_____ / _____*pertaining to*_____

Meaning: pertaining to the treatment of the seniors

1. hemolysis

   Elements _____ / _____ / _____
                    WR   CV   S

   Definitions _____ / _____ / _____

   Meaning:

2. antecubital

   Elements _____ / _____ / _____
                    P   WR   S

   Definitions _____ / _____ / _____

   Meaning:

3. subcutaneous

   Elements _____ / _____ / _____
                    P   WR   S

   Definitions _____ / _____ / _____

   Meaning:

4. hemodialysis

   Elements _____ / _____ / _____ / _____
                    WR   CV   WR   S

   Definitions _____ / _____ / _____ / _____

   Meaning:

5. venous

   Elements _____ / _____ / _____
                    P   WR   S

   Definitions _____ / _____ / _____

   Meaning:

6. pulmonary

   Elements _____ / _____ / _____
                    P   WR   S

   Definitions _____ / _____ / _____

   Meaning:

SKILLS DRILL 8-3: ROUTINE ETS VENIPUNCTURE (Text Procedure 8-2)

Fill in the blanks with the missing information.

Steps

1. Review and (1) _____ test request.

2. Approach, (5) _____, and prepare patient.

3. Verify (7) _____ restrictions and latex sensitivity.

4. Sanitize (10) _____ and put on gloves.

5. Position patient, apply tourniquet, and ask patient to make a (12) _____.

6. Select vein, (14) _____ _____, and ask patient to open fist.

Explanation/Rationale

A test request must be reviewed for completeness, date, and time of collection, status, and priority. The (2) _____ process records the request and assigns it a (3) _____ number used to (4) _____ the specimen, related processes, and paperwork.

The right approach for a successful patient encounter includes a professional bedside manner, being organized and efficient, and looking for signs that convey important inpatient information or infection-control precautions. Correct (6) _____ is vital to patient safety and meaningful test results. Name, DOB, and MR number must be verified and matched to the test order and inpatient's ID band. Preparing the patient by explaining procedures and addressing inquiries helps reduce patient anxiety.

Test results can be meaningless or (8) _____ and patient care (9) _____ if diet requirements have not been met. Exposure to latex can trigger a life-threatening reaction in those allergic to it.

Proper hand (11) _____ plays a major role in infection control by protecting the phlebotomist, patient, and others from contamination. Gloves are required by OSHA to protect the phlebotomist from bloodborne pathogen exposure.

Proper positioning is important to patient comfort and venipuncture success. The patient's arm should be placed downward in a straight line from shoulder to wrist to aid in vein selection and avoid reflux as tubes are filled. Tourniquet application enlarges veins and makes them easier to see, feel, and enter with a needle. A (13) _____ fist makes the veins easier to see and feel and helps keep them from rolling.

Select a large, well-anchored vein. The median cubital should be the first choice, followed by the cephalic. The (15) _____ should not be chosen unless it appears that no other vein can be safely or successfully accessed. Releasing the tourniquet and opening the fist helps prevent hemoconcentration.

7. Clean and (16) _____ site.

Cleaning the site with an antiseptic helps avoid contaminating the specimen or patient with skin-surface bacteria picked up by the needle during venipuncture. Letting the site (17) _____ naturally permits maximum antiseptic action, prevents contamination caused by wiping, and avoids stinging or burning on needle entry.

8. Prepare equipment.

Selecting appropriate equipment for the (18) _____, condition, and location of the vein is easier after vein selection. Preparing it while the site is drying saves time. Attach a needle to an ETS holder. Put the first tube in the holder now (see step 10) or wait until after needle entry. (19) _____ must be put on now if not already on.

9. Reapply tourniquet, uncap and
   (20) _____ needle.

The tourniquet aids needle entry. Pick up the tube holder with your dominant hand, placing your thumb on top near the needle end and fingers underneath. Uncap and (21) _____ the needle for (22) _____, and discard it if flawed.

10. Ask patient to remake a fist,
    (23) _____ vein, and insert needle.

The fist aids needle entry. (24) _____ stretches the skin, so the needle enters (25) _____ and with less pain, and keeps the vein from rolling.

Warn the patient. Line the needle up with the vein and insert it bevel up into the skin using a smooth forward motion. Stop when you feel a decrease in (26) _____, often described as a "pop," and press your fingers into the arm to anchor the holder.

11. Establish blood flow, release
    (27) _____, ask patient to open fist.

Blood will not flow until the needle pierces the tube stopper. Place a tube in the holder and push it partway onto the needle with a clockwise twist. Grasp the holder's flanges with your middle and index fingers, pulling back slightly to keep the holder from moving, and push the tube onto the needle with your thumb. Releasing the (28) _____ and opening the fist allows blood flow to normalize (see step 6). According to CLSI standards, the tourniquet should be released as soon as possible after blood begins to flow and should not be left on longer than 1 minute.

12. Fill, remove, and (29) _____ in order of draw.

Fill additive tubes until the vacuum is exhausted to ensure correct blood-to-additive ratio, and mix them (30) _____ upon removal from the holder using 3 to 8 gentle inversions (depending on type and manufacturer) to prevent clot formation. Follow the CLSI order of draw to prevent additive carryover between tubes.

13. Place gauze, remove needle, activate
    (31) _____ feature, and
    apply pressure.

A clean, folded gauze square is placed over the site, so pressure can be applied immediately after needle removal.

Remove the needle in one smooth motion without lifting up or pressing down on it. Immediately apply pressure to the site with your free hand while simultaneously activating the needle (32) _____ _____ with the other to prevent the chance of a needlestick.

14. Discard (33) _____
    _____.

According to OSHA, the needle and the (34) _____ _____ must go into the sharps container as a unit because removing a needle from the holder exposes the user to sharps injury.

15. (35) _____ _____.

To avoid mislabeling errors, label tubes before leaving the (36) _____ or dismissing the patient.

16. Observe special (37) _____
    instructions.

For accurate results, some specimens require special (38) _____ such as cooling in crushed ice (e.g., ammonia), transportation at (39) _____ temperature (e.g., cold agglutinin), or protection from (40) _____ (e.g., bilirubin).

17. Check (41) _____ _____
    and apply bandage

The patient's arm must be examined to verify that (42) _____ has stopped. The site must be checked for signs of bleeding beneath the skin. If bleeding has stopped, apply a bandage and advise the patient to keep it in place for at least 15 minutes. If bleeding persists beyond 5 minutes, notify the patient's nurse or physician.

18. Dispose of used and
    (43) _____
    materials

Materials such as needle caps and wrappers are normally discarded in the regular trash. Some facilities require that contaminated items such as blood-soaked gauze be discarded in (44) _____ containers.

19. Thank patient, remove gloves, and
    (45) _____ _____.

Thanking the patient is courteous and professional. Gloves must be removed in an aseptic manner and hands washed or (46) _____ with hand sanitizer as an infection-control precaution.

20. (47) _____ _____
to the lab.

Prompt delivery to the lab protects specimen (48) _____ and is typically achieved by personal delivery, transportation via a pneumatic tube system, or by a courier service.

SKILLS DRILL 8-4: USING A SYRINGE TRANSFER DEVICE (Text Procedure 8-5)

Fill in the blanks with the missing information.

Steps

1. Remove the (1) _____ from the syringe and discard it in a sharps container.

2. Attach the syringe (3) _____ to the transfer device hub, rotating it to ensure secure attachment.

3. Hold the syringe (5) _____ with the tip down and the transfer device at the bottom.

4. Place an ETS tube in the barrel of the transfer device and push it all the way (8) _____ _____ _____.

5. Follow the (10) _____ _____ _____ if multiple tubes are to be filled.

6. Keep the tubes and transfer device (13) _____.

7. Let tubes fill using the (17) _____ draw of the tube. Do not push on the (18) _____ _____.

8. If you must underfill a tube, (21) _____ _____ the plunger to stop blood flow before removing it.

9. (24) _____ additive tubes as soon as they are removed.

10. When finished, discard the syringe and transfer device (29) _____ in a sharps container.

Explanation/Rationale

The (2) _____ must be removed to attach the transfer device.

Secure attachment is necessary to prevent (4) _____ _____ during transfer.

This ensures (6) _____ placement of tubes to prevent (7) _____ _____.

The device has an internal (9) _____ that will puncture the stopper and allow blood to flow into the tube.

The (11) _____ _____ _____ is designed to prevent (12) _____ _____ between tubes.

This ensures that tubes fill from bottom to (14) _____, preventing additive (15) _____ with the needle and (16) _____ - _____ of subsequent tubes.

Forcing blood into a tube by pushing the (19) _____ can (20) _____ the specimen or cause the tube stopper to pop off, splashing tube contents.

Tubes quickly fill until the (22) _____ is gone. (23) _____ _____ the plunger stops the tube from filling.

(25) _____ tubes must be mixed (26) _____ for proper (27) _____, including preventing (28) _____ formation in anticoagulant tubes.

Removing the (30) _____ from the syringe would expose the user to (31) _____ in the hubs of both units. The transfer device must go into the sharps because of its internal (32) _____.

SKILLS DRILL 8-5: HIGHLIGHTS OF HAND VENIPUNCTURE PROCEDURE
(Text Procedure 8-3)

The following are highlights from the procedure for venipuncture of a hand vein using a butterfly and ETS holder. Fill in the blanks with the missing information.

1. Position Hand: Support the (A) _____ on the (B) _____ or armrest. Have the patient

   (C) _____ the fingers slightly or make a fist.

2. Select Vein: Select a vein that has (A) _____ or resilience and can be easily (B) _____.

   Wiping the hand with (C) _____ sometimes makes the veins more (D) _____.

3. Prepare Equipment: Attach the butterfly to an (A) _____. Grasp the (B) _____ near the

   needle end and run your fingers down its length, (C) _____ it slightly to help keep it from

   (D) _____ _____ ___.

4. Uncap and Inspect Needle: Hold the (A) _____ portion of the butterfly between your

   (B) _____ and index finger or fold the wings upright and grasp them together. Cradle the tubing

   and holder in the (C) _____ of your dominant hand or lay it next to the patient's hand. Uncap and

   inspect the needle for (D) _____ and discard it if flawed.

5. Anchor the vein: Anchoring (A) _____ the (B) _____ so the needle enters easily and with

   less (C) _____ and it keeps the vein from (D) _____.

6. Insert the Needle: Insert the needle into the vein at a shallow angle of approximately (A) _____

   degrees or less. A (B) "_____" or small amount of (C) _____ will appear in the

   (D) _____ when the needle is in the vein. "Seat" the needle by slightly threading it within the

   (E) _____ of the vein to keep it from twisting back out of the vein if you let go of it.

7. Establish Blood Flow: The (A) _____ of blood in the (B) _____ indicates vein

   (C) _____. Blood will not flow until the needle pierces the tube (D) _____. Place a tube

   in the holder and push it part way onto the needle with a clockwise twist. Grasp the holder

   (E) _____ with your middle and index fingers, pulling back slightly to keep the (F) _____

   from moving, and push the tube onto the needle with your thumb.

8. Fill, Remove, and Mix Tubes: Maintain tubing and holder (A) _____ the site, and positioned, so that

   the tubes fill from the (B) _____ to prevent (C) _____.

SKILLS DRILL 8-6: HIGHLIGHTS OF NEEDLE-AND-SYRINGE VENIPUNCTURE PROCEDURE (Text Procedure 8-4)

The following are highlights from the needle-and-syringe venipuncture procedure. Fill in the blanks with the missing information.

1. Prepare Equipment: It is easier to select (A) _____ equipment after the (B) _____ has

   been chosen. Preparing it while the site is (C) _____ saves time.

2. Uncap and Inspect Needle: Hold the syringe in your dominant hand as you would an (A)_____

   (B) _____. Place your (C) _____ on top near the needle end and fingers underneath.

   Uncap and (D) _____ the needle for defects and discard it if flawed.

3. Establish Blood Flow: Establishment of blood flow is normally indicated by (A) _____ in the

   (B) _____ of the syringe. In some cases blood will not flow until the syringe

   (C) _____ is (D) _____ (E) _____.

4. Fill Syringe: Venous blood will not automatically (A) _____ (B) _____ a syringe. It must

   be filled by slowly pulling back on the (C) _____ with your free hand. Steady the syringe as you

   would an (D) _____ (E) _____ during routine venipuncture.

5. Discard Needle: The needle must be removed and discarded in the sharps container, so that a

   (A) _____ device for (B) _____ the tubes can be (C) _____ to the syringe. A

   (D) _____ device greatly reduces the chance of accidental (E) _____ (F) _____

   and confines any (G) _____ or spraying that may be generated as the tube is removed.

Crossword

ACROSS

1. Meaning of AC
4. Order stating not to revive (plural)
6. Preferred is 30 degrees or less
8. To secure firmly by pulling the skin taut
10. Closed blood collection system (abbrev.)
13. Applied to sample tube after collection, never before (plural)
14. To use an alcohol-based cleansing solution
15. Pertaining to veins or blood passing through them
17. Median cutaneous _____
19. Alcohol used in routine venipuncture
21. Intensive care unit (abbrev.)
22. Vein status that requires the use of small-gauge needle and syringe
24. Pulled tight
26. Assigned number to each patient (abbrev.)
27. Equipment checked for imperfections/burrs before puncturing
28. Used instead of cotton ball over the puncture hole
30. Location of preferred choice of veins for venipuncture (abbrev.)
31. State of not eating
33. Tight hand used to stabilize veins in the arm
34. To thread the needle within the lumen
35. Basilic and cephalic
36. Identification (abbrev.)
37. Type of dialysis

DOWN

1. Another name for ID bracelet
2. Former recommended way to swipe a swab to clean the site
3. Type of glove and tourniquet responsible for allergenic reactions
5. Used to relay patient status and usually posted on the door (plural)
7. Topical anesthetic applied to skin to ease puncture pain
9. Type of care for patients who are terminally ill
11. Pink- to red-colored plasma is due to
_____
12. Point at which the needle will enter the vein
15. Type of gloves used for venipuncture
16. Layer of connective and adipose tissue below the dermis
18. Backflow of blood from collection tube to patient's vein
19. The most important part of venipuncture procedure is to _____ the patient
20. One who is receiving medical care
23. Pertaining to elderly patients
25. Test commonly ordered on geriatric patients if RA is suspected (abbrev.)
28. Nitrile or vinyl _____
29. Prescribed course of eating and drinking
32. National Institute on Aging (abbrev.)

Chapter Review Questions

1. A vein that has patency
   a. feels hard and cord like.
   b. has a bounce or resilience to it.
   c. is fairly deep in the tissues.
   d. should not be used for venipuncture.

2. Which type of test requisition has been shown to decrease laboratory errors?
   a. Bar coded
   b. Computer
   c. Manual
   d. Verbal

3. The time is 07:50 hours. You have received the following test requests on different patients. Which test specimen should you collect first?
   a. CBC ordered ASAP
   b. Cortisol ordered for 08:00
   c. Fasting glucose
   d. Postop hemoglobin

4. A student asks the patient for permission to draw a blood specimen. Which of the following answers implies that the student does not really have permission?
   a. As long as you're good at it.
   b. Which arm do you want?
   c. Yes, but I would rather not.
   d. All of the above.

5. You have a request to collect a stat specimen. A doctor is with the patient when you arrive. What should you do?
   a. Call your supervisor and ask what you should do.
   b. Excuse yourself and politely ask the doctor if you can do the draw.
   c. Leave the room and return when the doctor is gone.
   d. Stand there quietly until the doctor sees you and asks what you want.

6. You are in the process of identifying an inpatient. The patient's verbal confirmation of name and date of birth matches the requisition, but the medical record number is different. What should you do?
   a. Change the requisition number to match the ID band and collect the specimen.
   b. Collect the specimen and inform the patient's nurse that the ID needs correcting.
   c. Do not collect the specimen until the problem has been addressed and resolved.
   d. Fill out an incident report and return to the lab without collecting the specimen.

7. You are a phlebotomy student on rotation at an outpatient site. A patient who seems extremely apprehensive about having her blood drawn tells you that she is afraid of needles. What should you do?
   a. Ask an experienced phlebotomist to perform the draw for you.
   b. Explain to her that you will use a small needle that barely hurts.
   c. Tell her that it is not a big deal and that she shouldn't be afraid.
   d. Use an ice pack to numb the site before drawing the specimen.

8. There are two patients in a room. One of them has a latex allergy. You have a request to collect a blood specimen on the other one. How should you proceed?
   a. Ask the allergic patient to wear a mask until you leave.
   b. Do not take anything that contains latex into the room.
   c. Pull the curtain between the beds and proceed normally.
   d. Your patient is not allergic to latex, so proceed as usual.

9. The best way to judge patency of a vein is to
   a. feel it to determine the strength of the pulse.
   b. palpate above and below where you first feel it.
   c. press and release it several times to determine resilience.
   d. roll your finger from side to side while pressing against it.

10. Which of the following statements describes proper venipuncture technique?
    a. Clean the site quickly while the tourniquet is on.
    b. Fill additive tubes until the vacuum is exhausted.
    c. Keep the tourniquet on until the last tube is full.
    d. Wipe the alcohol dry to prevent it from stinging.

11. What is the most critical error a phlebotomist can make?
    a. Collecting a timed specimen late
    b. Failing to collect a specimen
    c. Giving a patient a hematoma
    d. Misidentifying a patient specimen

12. Which needle can be removed from the blood collection unit before disposal?
    a. Butterfly needle
    c. Syringe needle
    b. ETS needle
    d. None of the above

13. When should additive tubes be mixed?
    a. After all the other tubes have been collected.
    b. As soon as they are removed from the holder.
    c. Never. Additive tubes do not require mixing.
    d. While you are filling any of the other tubes.

14. You have made two unsuccessful attempts while trying to collect an ASAP specimen on an inpatient. The specimen cannot be collected by skin puncture. What should you do next?
    a. Ask another phlebotomist to collect it.
    b. Ask the patient's nurse to do the draw.
    c. Collect it by arterial puncture.
    d. Try to draw it one more time.

15. The proper way to transfer blood from a syringe into an ETS tube is to
    a. discard the needle, open the tube, and slowly eject the blood into it.
    b. hold the tube carefully and insert the needle through the tube stopper.
    c. place the tube in a rack and insert the needle through the tube stopper.
    d. safely remove the needle and attach a transfer device to fill the tube.

16. How can you tell that you are in a vein when drawing blood with a butterfly?
    a. Engage the tube to see if it will fill.
    b. Blood usually appears in the tubing.
    c. You can hear a soft popping sound.
    d. There is no easy way you can tell.

17. You are performing a venipuncture on a difficult vein using a butterfly. You have an SST and a light-blue–top tube to collect. How do you proceed?
    a. Collect and mix the SST before filling and mixing the light-blue top.
    b. Collect and mix the light-blue top before filling and mixing the SST.
    c. Draw a clear tube, fill and mix the light-blue top, then fill and mix the SST.
    d. Draw half the SST, then fill and mix the light-blue top, then finish the SST.

18. Interventions to ease pain in collecting blood specimens from infants include
    a. EMLA.
    c. pacifiers.
    b. oral sucrose.
    d. all of the above.

19. Skin changes in elderly patients can make it harder to
    a. anchor veins.
    c. palpate veins.
    b. injure veins.
    d. see the veins.

20. Which type of disease is most likely to cause tremors?
    a. Alzheimer
    c. Diabetes
    b. Arthritis
    d. Parkinson

Case Studies

Case Study 8-1: Patient ID and Specimen Labeling

A phlebotomist received a verbal request for a stat blood draw in the ER. When he arrived the nurse told him that the patient (Mr. Johnson) was in bed 1 and needed electrolytes and an H&H drawn. The patient had no ID band. The nurse assured the phlebotomist that it was the correct patient and that she would prepare the requisition and labels while he drew the specimens. The patient was able to verbally confirm name and date of birth, so the phlebotomist proceeded to collect the specimens, a green top and a lavender top. Just as he was finishing up, the nurse told the phlebotomist that they had another stat draw in bed 3. This patient needed electrolytes and glucose specimens drawn. The nurse said that she hadn't had time to prepare the requisition or labels for either patient, but she would do so now. The phlebotomist put the first two specimens in his phlebotomy tray and headed for bed 3. This patient was unconscious, and no one else was there to confirm his identity. The nurse said she didn't know his name either, as he had no identification with him when he was found. The phlebotomist proceeded to collect the specimens, a green top and a lavender top, as with the first patient. He put the specimens in the tray when he was finished and went to the nurses' station for the requisitions and labels, which the nurse did have ready for him. When he went to label the specimens he had to stop and think about which specimens were the correct ones for each patient since they were the same type of tubes. He was pretty sure he had put each patient's specimens at opposite ends of the tray, but had he turned the tray around since then? He decided that the ones that felt warmest were the last ones drawn, placed the labels on the tubes, and delivered them to the lab.

QUESTIONS

1. The phlebotomist made several errors. What were they?

2. What should the phlebotomist have done differently to prevent each error?

3. How might the actions of the phlebotomist affect treatment of the patients?

Case Study 8-2: Blood Volume, Equipment Selection, and Syringe Transfer Technique

A phlebotomist must collect specimens for a PTT and a CBC on an infant. The infant is several months old but was born prematurely and weighs only 5 pounds. The phlebotomist is surprised to see that the infant has a prominent median cubital vein. He uses a 10-mL syringe and a 23-gauge butterfly needle and is able to collect about 5 mL of blood before the tiny vein blows and a hematoma starts to form. He withdraws the needle and quickly bandages the site. He uses a transfer device to deliver the required 4.5 mL into a light-blue–top tube for the PTT. He then uses a 5-mL syringe to draw another 5 mL of blood from a vein in the infant's other arm. He then discovers that he does not have another transfer device, so he grabs the lavender top and attempts to insert the needle through the tube stopper. The needle slips and jabs his hand. He is bleeding badly, so he drops the tube and syringe into his phlebotomy tray and runs to the sink to wash the wound. He then wraps a paper towel around his hand and returns to fill the lavender-top tube. This time he removes the needle from the syringe and the stopper from the tube. He injects the blood into the tube and replaces the stopper. He labels both tubes and returns to the lab. Specimen processing ultimately rejects both specimens, the PTT because of hemolysis and the CBC because of clotting.

QUESTIONS

1. What is the infant's estimated blood volume and calculated blood volume? How many milliliters of blood would be 10% of each of these numbers?

2. Was it appropriate to collect 10 mL of blood from the infant for the two tests? Why or why not?

3. How could the phlebotomist have collected less blood for the required tests?

4. How could the phlebotomist have avoided injury?

5. What could have caused the hemolysis of the PTT and the clotting of the CBC?

Case Study 8-3: Drawing Blood from a Transplant Patient

George, a phlebotomist has a bilirubin and ammonia to collect on a patient on the transplant floor in the surgical intensive care unit. It is his last of the morning draws and he is anxious to get back to the lab. He has plans to meet a friend on his coffee break. A nurse is just leaving the patient's room. She says she will be back in a minute to assist. George waits a few minutes, but the nurse does not return. He can't imagine why she would need to assist him with anything, so he decides to go ahead with the draw. The patient is semiawake and mumbles his name when George verifies his identification. George finds a vein and starts to insert the needle. Suddenly the patient jerks his arm away. George almost sticks himself with the needle and quickly activates the needle safety device. Blood is running down the patient's arm and George tries to hold gauze over it but the patient thrashes about. The nurse comes rushing into the room. She is mad at George for not waiting for her. She calms the patient down, holds his arm steady and George is able to collect the specimens. George then grabs his tray and the tubes and heads back to the lab, labeling and initialing the tubes on his way.

QUESTIONS

1. What do you think made the patient so combative?

2. What should George have done differently?

3. George did not handle the specimens correctly. What did he fail to do?

Chapter 9
Preanalytical Considerations

Objectives

Study the information in your TEXTBOOK that corresponds to each objective to prepare yourself for the activities in this chapter.

1 Demonstrate basic knowledge of the preanalytical variables that influence laboratory test results, define associated terminology, and identify the tests most affected by each one.

2 Discuss problem areas associated with site selection including various vascular access sites and devices, and explain what to do when they are encountered.

3 Describe how to handle patient complications and conditions pertaining to blood collection, address procedural error risks, and specimen quality concerns, and analyze reasons for failure to draw blood.

Matching

Use choices only once unless otherwise indicated.

MATCHING 9-1: KEY TERMS AND DESCRIPTIONS

Match each key term with the *best* description.

Key Terms (1–16)

1. _____ A-line
2. _____ AV shunt/fistula/graft
3. _____ Bariatric
4. _____ Basal state
5. _____ Bilirubin
6. _____ CVAD
7. _____ CVC
8. _____ Diurnal/circadian
9. _____ Edema
10. _____ Exsanguination
11. _____ Hematoma
12. _____ Hemoconcentration
13. _____ Hemolysis
14. _____ Iatrogenic
15. _____ Icteric
16. _____ Implanted port

Descriptions

A. Abnormal accumulation of fluid in the tissues
B. Blood loss to the point where life cannot be sustained
C. Catheter placed in an artery, most commonly the radial
D. Central vascular access device or indwelling line
E. Central venous catheter or central venous line
F. Decreased blood fluid and increase in nonfilterable components
G. Destruction of RBCs and release of hemoglobin into blood fluid
H. Happening daily, or having a 24-hour cycle
I. Product of the breakdown of RBCs
J. Relating to the treatment of obesity
K. Resting state of the body in early AM after a 12-hour fast
L. Small chamber placed under the skin usually in the upper chest
M. Surgical joining of an artery and vein
N. Swelling or mass of blood caused by blood leaking from a blood vessel
O. Term used to describe a specimen marked by jaundice
P. Term that describes an adverse condition due to treatment

Key Terms (17–31)

17. _____ IV
18. _____ Jaundice
19. _____ Lipemic
20. _____ Lymphostasis
21. _____ Petechiae
22. _____ PICC
23. _____ Preanalytical
24. _____ Reference ranges
25. _____ Reflux
26. _____ Saline lock
27. _____ Sclerosed
28. _____ Syncope
29. _____ Thrombosed
30. _____ Vasovagal
31. _____ Venous stasis

Descriptions

A. Backflow of blood into the vein during venipuncture
B. Catheter with a stopcock or cap for delivering medication
C. Clotted, or denoting a vessel containing a clot
D. Fainting
E. Hard, cord-like, and lacking resilience
F. Icterus, a condition characterized by increased bilirubin
G. Normal laboratory test values for healthy individuals
H. Peripherally inserted central catheter
I. Prior to analysis
J. Relating to the action of a particular nerve on blood vessels
K. Stagnation or stoppage of the normal blood flow
L. Stoppage or obstruction of normal lymph flow
M. Term that describes serum or plasma that has a milky look
N. Tiny, nonraised red or purple spots on patient's skin
O. Within, or pertaining to the inside of a vein

MATCHING 9-2: PHYSIOLOGICAL EFFECT AND TEST

Match the physiological effect to the associated test.

Physiological Effect

1. _____ Crying can increase levels

2. _____ Decreases with age

3. _____ Dehydration increases levels

4. _____ Elevated levels are related to jaundice

5. _____ Fatty foods increase levels

6. _____ Fever causes levels to increase

7. _____ Increases with altitude

8. _____ Levels increase with pancreatitis caused by steroid use

9. _____ Levels normally peak around 08:00 hours

10. _____ Requires documentation of patient's position during collection

11. _____ Smoking decreases levels

12. _____ Stays elevated for 24 hours or more after exercise

Test

A. Amylase
B. Bilirubin
C. CK
D. Coagulation factors
E. Cortisol
F. Creatinine clearance
G. IgA
H. Insulin
I. Lipids
J. Plasma renin
K. RBC count
L. WBC count

MATCHING 9-3: PROBLEM SITE AND DRAWBACK

Match the problem venipuncture site to the possible drawback if a blood specimen is collected from it.

Problem Site

1. _____ Arm with a large hematoma

2. _____ Edematous arm

3. _____ Mastectomy on that side of the body

4. _____ Obese arm

5. _____ Paralyzed arm

6. _____ Recently burned antecubital area

7. _____ Tattoo-covered arm

8. _____ Vein that feels sclerosed

Drawback

A. Could mean veins are deeper than normal
B. Freshly dyed areas could be easily infected
C. Impaired circulation could affect test results
D. Increased risk of thrombosis
E. Results could be affected by lymphostasis
F. Site may be painful and susceptible to infection
G. Skin could be injured by tourniquet application
H. Specimen could be contaminated by hemolyzed blood

MATCHING 9-4: SCENARIOS AND VASCULAR ACCESS DEVICES

Match the type of equipment described in the following scenarios with the list of vascular access devices.

Scenarios

1. _____ A nurse is collecting a blood gas specimen from tubing inserted in the underside of a patient's left wrist on the thumb side.

2. _____ A nurse is palpating an area in the patient's upper chest. She tells the patient that she is looking for the "chamber."

3. _____ A patient in the dialysis unit has what appears to be a loop under the skin on the inside of his forearm in which the large needles connected to the dialysis tubing have been inserted.

4. _____ There are several short lengths of capped tubing protruding from a patient's left arm, just above the antecubital area.

5. _____ There is a device inserted on the back of a patient's arm just above the wrist. The device has a thin, rubber-like cover through which a nurse is administering fluid from a syringe.

6. _____ The patient is a line draw. He has three short lengths of capped tubing protruding from his chest. The nurse draws the specimen for you from one of the lengths of tubing.

Vascular Access Devices

A. Arterial line (A-line)
B. Arteriovenous (AV) shunt
C. Central venous catheter (CVC)
D. Implanted port
E. Peripherally inserted central catheter (PICC)
F. Saline lock

MATCHING 9-5: RISK AND PROCEDURAL ERROR

Match the risk to the procedural error involved.

Risk

1. _____ Hematoma formation

2. _____ Iatrogenic anemia

3. _____ Inadvertent arterial puncture

4. _____ Infection

5. _____ Nerve damage

6. _____ Reflux

7. _____ Vein damage

Procedural Error

A. A patient is a difficult draw, so the phlebotomist uses the exact same site each time.
B. Blood fills the stopper end of the tube first.
C. Blood spurts into the tube after the needle is redirected multiple times.
D. The needle goes through the vein.
E. The patient complains of great pain during a missed attempt to draw from the basilic vein.
F. The phlebotomist always wipes the alcohol dry before performing a venipuncture.
G. Three 5-mL tubes of blood are drawn from an infant at one time.

MATCHING 9-6: SENTENCE BEGINNING AND ENDING (Text Box 9-3)

Match the beginning of the sentence concerning causes of hemolysis with the letter of the correct sentence ending.

Sentence Beginning

1. Drawing blood through a _____
2. Failure to wipe away the first drop of _____
3. Forceful aspiration of _____
4. Forcing the blood _____
5. Frothing of blood _____
6. Horizontal transport of _____
7. Mixing additive tubes _____
8. Partially filling a _____
9. Pulling back the _____
10. Rough handling _____
11. Squeezing the site _____
12. Syringe transfer _____
13. Using a large volume _____
14. Using a needle with a _____

Sentence Ending

A. blood during a syringe draw
B. capillary blood, which can contain alcohol residue
C. caused by improper fit of the needle on a syringe
D. delay in which partially clotted blood is forced into a tube
E. during capillary specimen collection
F. during transport
G. from a syringe into an evacuated tube
H. hematoma
I. normal draw sodium fluoride tube
J. plunger too quickly during a syringe draw
K. diameter that is too small for venipuncture
L. tube with a small-diameter butterfly needle
M. tubes, which let the blood slosh back and forth
N. vigorously, shaking them, or inverting them too quickly or forcefully

Labeling Exercises

LABELING EXERCISE 9-1: IDENTIFYING VENIPUNCTURE PROBLEMS

One of the following illustrations shows correct needle position. The other illustrations depict venipuncture problems. For each illustration, identify the problem depicted and write it (or correct needle position, if applicable) on the line beneath the illustration, followed by the letter of the corrective action required from the list below. Choices may be used more than once.

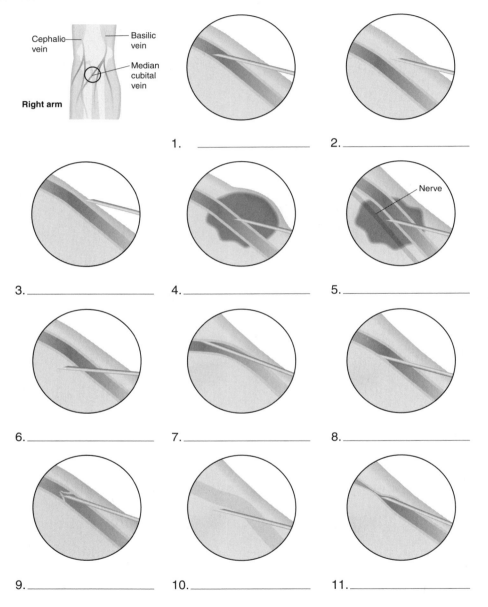

1. _____   2. _____

3. _____   4. _____   5. _____

6. _____   7. _____   8. _____

9. _____   10. _____   11. _____

Corrective Action

A. No corrective action required.
B. Discontinue the draw.
C. Disengage the tube, pull the needle back slightly, and re-engage the tube.
D. Disengage the tube, pull the needle back until only the bevel is under the skin, anchor the vein, redirect the needle, and re-engage the tube.

E. Gently push the needle forward.
F. Put on a new tube.
G. Try using a smaller-volume tube.
H. Withdraw the needle slowly until blood flow is obtained.

LABELING EXERCISE 9-2: VAD IDENTIFICATION

The following are examples of VAD placement in patients. Identify and label each one by writing the type of VAD on the line beneath it. Use the VAD full name and initials if applicable.

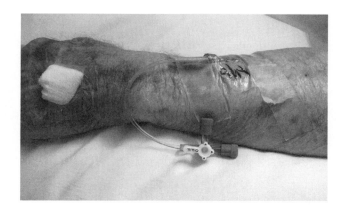

1. _____

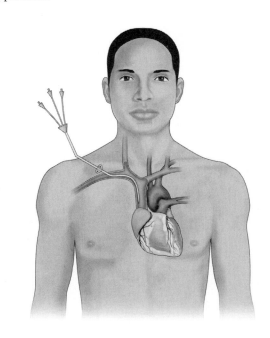

2. _____

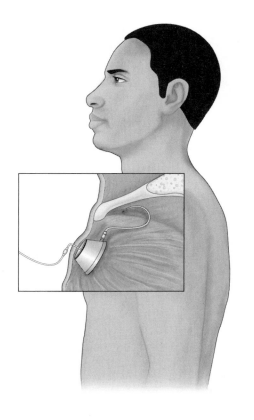

3. _____

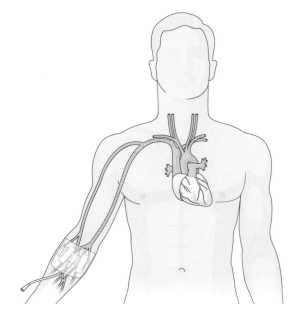

4. _____

Knowledge Drills

KNOWLEDGE DRILL 9-1: CAUTION AND KEY POINT RECOGNITION

The following sentences are from "CAUTION and KEY POINT" statements found throughout Chapter 9 of the TEXTBOOK. Using the TEXTBOOK, fill in the blanks with the missing information.

1. The National Cholesterol Education Program recommends that (A) _____ profiles be collected in a consistent manner after the patient has been either (B) _____ or _____ quietly for a minimum of (C) _____ _____.

2. Never apply a (A) _____ _____ _____ or (B) _____, or perform venipuncture, on an arm with any type of (C) _____.

3. Do not use (A) _____ _____ to revive patients who have fainted as they can have unwanted side effects such as (B) _____ distress in (C) _____ individuals.

4. If you sense that the patient is in pain, or the patient complains of (A) _____ or _____ pain, or asks you to remove the (B) _____ for any reason, the venipuncture should be (C) _____ immediately, even if there are no other signs of (D) _____ _____.

5. Extreme pain, a burning or (A)_____ _____ sensation, (B) _____ of the arm, and pain that radiates up or down the arm are all signs of (C) _____ involvement, and any one of them requires immediate (D) _____ of the venipuncture.

6. Hand or fist (A) _____ can (B) _____ blood (C) _____ levels up to 20%.

7. _____ is painful to the patient and can cause tears in the vein wall that result in (B) _____ formation, damage (C) _____ and other tissues, or lead to inadvertent puncture of an (D) _____.

8. Although there are a number of different causes, jaundice in a patient may indicate (A) _____ inflammation caused by (B) _____ B or C (C) _____.

9. To ensure collection of noncontaminated blood, never perform venipuncture through a (A) _____. If there is no alternative site, perform the venipuncture (B) _____ to the (C) _____ to ensure the collection of (D) _____-_____ blood.

10. Only (A) _____ and other specially (B) _____ personnel are allowed to draw blood specimens from (C) _____ _____ _____ (_____).

11. Never apply a (A) _____ _____ instead of maintaining pressure until bleeding has stopped, and do not (B) _____ an outpatient or (C) _____ an inpatient until bleeding has stopped or the appropriate personnel have taken charge of the situation.

12. A rapidly forming (A) _____ may indicate that an (B) _____ has been (C) _____ hit.

KNOWLEDGE DRILL 9-2: SCRAMBLED WORDS

Unscramble the following words using the hints given in parentheses and the letters that have been placed in the correct boxes. Finish writing the correct spelling of the scrambled words in the corresponding boxes.

1. ajecudin (could indicate hepatitis)

   | | | u | | | | c | |

2. cemhootninecronat (an indirect result of venous stasis)

   | | | m | o | | | n | | | | | a | | | | |

3. ecepahiet (a sign that the site may bleed excessively)

   | p | | | | | | i | | |

4. oratiecing (as a result of treatment)

   | | a | | | | | e | | | |

5. polsecdal (describes a vein that has shut down)

   | | | l | l | | | | | |

6. psoynec (patient reaction to fear of venipuncture)

   | | | | c | o | | |

7. rudalin (happening daily)

   | d | | | | | | l |

8. sblaa (type of metabolic state)

   | | | s | | |

9. smettmycoa (issues with this side for a blood draw)

   | | a | | | e | | t | | | |

10. soyiteb (could lead to difficult arm draws)

    | | b | | | | y | |

11. thrandeoyid (decrease in total body fluid)

    | | | h | | d | | | | | | |

12. xuferl (proper arm position helps avoid this)

    | | | | | | x | |

KNOWLEDGE DRILL 9-3: TRUE/FALSE ACTIVITY

The following statements are all false. Circle the one or two words that make the statement false and write the correct word(s) that would make the statement true in the space provided.

1. The preanalytical phase of the testing process begins for the laboratory when the specimen is analyzed.

2. One way a physician evaluates a patient's test results is by comparing them to previous results on other patients.

3. Lipemia can be present for up to 8 hours, which is why accurate testing of triglycerides requires an 8-hour fast.

4. It is recommended that CK and LDH levels be drawn after intramuscular injections.

5. Jaundice in a patient may indicate liver inflammation caused by the herpes virus.

6. A fistula is a temporary surgical connection of an artery and vein.

7. Avoid edematous areas for blood draw because the veins are harder to locate, and you will find the tissue is scarred.

8. Blood specimens should not be collected from a known previous IV site within 12 to 18 hours of the time the IV was discontinued.

9. A procedural error that can cause specimen hemolysis is transporting tubes vertically.

10. One of the ways a phlebotomist can get blood from a vein that has collapsed is to remove the tourniquet.

11. Nerve injury can occur from improper vein selection or inserting the needle too superficially.

12. When an outpatient who has fainted regains consciousness, he or she must remain in the area for at least 5 minutes.

KNOWLEDGE DRILL 9-4: HEMATOMA FORMATION (Text Box 9-1)

The following are six situations that can trigger hematoma formation. Fill in the blanks with the missing information.

1. The vein is _____ for the needle size.

2. The needle penetrates _____.

3. The needle is _____ into the vein.

4. Excessive or _____ is used to locate the vein.

5. The needle is removed while the _____.

6. _____ is not adequately applied following venipuncture.

7. _____ to hold the gauze in place after venipuncture.

8. _____ is accidently punctured.

KNOWLEDGE DRILL 9-5: IATROGENIC BLOOD LOSS

List four ways to minimize iatrogenic blood loss.

1. _____

2. _____

3. _____

4. _____

KNOWLEDGE DRILL 9-6: HEMOCONCENTRATION

Place a "C" in front of each sentence that describes an action that causes hemoconcentration. Place a "P" in front of each sentence that describes an action that prevents hemoconcentration.

1. _____ Allowing the patient to pump the fist

2. _____ Asking the patient to release the fist upon blood flow

3. _____ Choosing an appropriate patent vein

4. _____ Excessively massaging the area when locating a vein

5. _____ Redirecting the needle multiple times in search of a vein

6. _____ Releasing the tourniquet within 1 minute

KNOWLEDGE DRILL 9-7: SERUM APPEARANCE

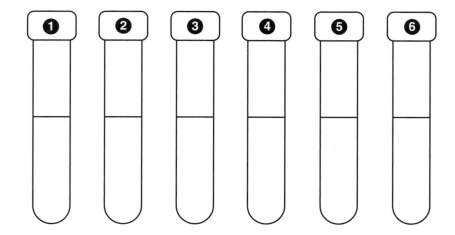

Color the serum in the numbered aliquot tubes according to the appearance listed by tube number below.

Serum Appearance

1. Icteric
2. Lipemic
3. Mild hemolysis
4. Moderate hemolysis
5. Gross hemolysis
6. Normal

Skills Drills

SKILLS DRILL 9-1: REQUISITION ACTIVITY

Instructions: Answer the following questions concerning the test requisition shown below.

1. Identify two physiological variables that affect Hgb levels and identify the effect. _____

2. If this patient's bilirubin level is high, how might it affect the patient's appearance, and why? _____

_____

3. How will the phlebotomist obtain this specimen? _____

4. Identify the tube required for each test. _____

_____

Any Hospital USA
1123 West Physician Drive
Any Town USA

Laboratory Test Requisition

- -

PATIENT INFORMATION:

Name: _____Smith_____Jane_____R_____
            (last)   (first)   (MI)

Identification Number: __09365784_____ Birth Date: __06/21/63__

Referring Physician: __Coleman_____

Date to be Collected: __03/11/2015_____ Time to be Collected: __0600____

Special Instructions: __Line draw only_____

- -

TEST(S) REQUIRED:

_____ NH4 – Ammonia	_____ Gluc – glucose
__X__ Bili – Bilirubin, total & direct	__X__ Hgb – hemoglobin
_____ BMP – basic metabolic panel	_____ Lact – lactic acid/lactate
_____ BUN – Blood urea nitrogen	_____ Plt. Ct. – platelet count
_____ Lytes – electrolytes	_____ PT – prothrombin time
_____ CBC – complete blood count	_____ PTT – partial thromboplastin time
_____ Chol – cholesterol	_____ RPR – rapid plasma reagin
_____ ESR – erythrocyte sed rate	_____ T&S – type and screen
_____ EtOH – alcohol	_____ PSA – prostate specific antigen
_____ D-dimer	Other _____

SKILLS DRILL 9-2: WORD BUILDING

Divide each of the words below into all of its elements (parts); prefix (P), word root (WR), combining vowel (CV), and suffix (S). Write the word part and its definition on the corresponding lines. Write the general meaning of the word in the space provided. If the word does not have a particular element, write NA (not applicable) in its place.

Example: Lymphostasis

Elements ____NA____ / ____lymph____ / ____o____ / ____stasis____

                      P   WR   CV   S

Definitions _____ / ____lymph____ / _____ / ____stopping____

Meaning: stopping lymph flow

1. Arteriovenous

   Elements _____ / _____ / _____ / _____ / _____

                     WR   CV   WR   S

   Definitions _____ / _____ / _____ / _____ / _____

   Meaning:

2. Bariatric

   Elements _____ / _____ / _____ / _____ / _____

                     WR   CV   S   S

   Definitions _____ / _____ / _____ / _____ / _____

3. Hemolysis

   Elements _____ / _____ / _____ / _____ / _____

                     P   WR   CV   S

   Definitions _____ / _____ / _____ / _____ / _____

   Meaning:

4. Intravenous

   Elements _____ / _____ / _____ / _____ / _____

                     P   WR   CV   S

   Definitions _____ / _____ / _____ / _____ / _____

   Meaning:

5. Lipemia

   Elements _____ / _____ / _____ / _____ / _____

                     P   WR   CV   S

   Definitions _____ / _____ / _____ / _____ / _____

   Meaning:

6. Sclerosis

   Elements _____ / _____ / _____ / _____ / _____

                     P   WR   CV   S

   Definitions _____ / _____ / _____ / _____ / _____

   Meaning:

7. Venostasis

   Elements _____ / _____ / _____ / _____ / _____

                     P   WR   CV   S

   Definitions _____ / _____ / _____ / _____ / _____

   Meaning:

SKILLS DRILL 9-3: VENIPUNCTURE BELOW AN IV (Text Procedure 9-1)

Fill in the blanks with the missing information.

Steps

1. Ask the patient's nurse to turn off the IV for at least (A) _____ prior to collection.

2. Apply the tourniquet (D) _____ to the IV.

3. Select a venipuncture site (F) _____ to the IV and the tourniquet.

4. Perform the venipuncture in a (J) _____ _____ than the one with the IV if possible.

5. Ask the nurse to (M) _____ after the specimen has been collected.

6. Document that the specimen was collected (P) _____ an IV, indicate the (Q) _____ in the IV, and identify which (R) _____

Explanation/Rationale

A phlebotomist is not qualified to make IV (B) _____. Turning off the IV for (C) _____ allows IV fluids to dissipate from the area. Avoids (E) _____ the IV.

Venous blood flows up the arm (G) _____ _____. Drawing (H) _____ an IV affords the best chance of obtaining blood that is free of (I) _____.

IV fluids can be present (K) _____ because of (L) _____ and may still be there after the IV is shut off because of poor venous circulation. IV flow rates must be (N) _____, and starting or adjusting them is not part of a phlebotomist's (O) _____.

This aids (S) _____ _____ and the patient's physician in the event that (T) _____ are questioned.

SKILLS DRILL 9-4: FAINTING PROCEDURE (Procedure 9-2)

Fill in the blanks with the missing information.

Steps

1. Release the (A) _____ and remove and discard the needle as quickly and safely as possible.

2. Apply pressure to the site while having the patient lower the (D) _____ and breathe deeply.

3. (G) _____ to the patient.

4. Physically (J) _____ the patient.

5. Ask (M) _____ and explain what you are doing if it is necessary to loosen a tight collar or tie.

6. Apply a (P) _____ compress or wet washcloth to the (Q) _____ and back of the _____.

7. Have someone stay with the patient until (S) _____ is complete.

8. Call (V) _____ personnel if the patient does not respond.

9. (X) _____ the incident according to facility protocol.

Explanation/Rationale

Discontinuing the draw and safely discarding the needle protects the (B) _____ and _____ from (C) _____ should the patient faint.

Pressure must be applied to prevent bleeding or bruising. Lowering the (E) _____ and breathing deeply helps get oxygenated blood to the (F) _____.

Diverts patient's attention, helps keep the patient (H) _____, and aids in assessing the patient's (I) _____.

Prevents (K) _____ in case of (L) _____.

Avoids (N) _____ of actions that are standard (O) _____ to hasten recovery.

Is thought to (R) _____ _____.

Prevents patient from (T) _____ too soon and possibly causing (U) _____-_____.

Emergency medicine is not in the phlebotomist's (W) _____ of _____.

(Y) _____ issues could arise and (Z) _____ is essential at that time.

Crossword

ACROSS

1. Result of damaged RBCs
4. Another name for indwelling line (abbrev.)
7. Possible result of mastectomy
9. Medical term for fainting
10. Having a 24-hour cycle
12. Describes blood loss due to testing
13. Broviac or Hickman (abbrev.)
14. Surgical connection of an artery and a vein
16. Excess tissue fluid
17. Describes a clotted vein
20. Increased temperature
21. Resting metabolic state
24. Intravenous line (abbrev.)
25. Fusion of an artery and a vein
27. Arteriovenous (abbrev.)
29. Trauma-related complication
30. Usually precedes vomiting
31. Preferred _____ is "fasting"
33. Phlebotomy national standards
34. Distinct buzzing VAD sensation
35. To clear a catheter with saline

DOWN

1. Result of decreased plasma volume
2. Extreme chubbiness
3. Brand of elastic pressure wrap
5. Cephalic or basilic
6. Pertaining to increased bilirubin
8. Disease caused by HIV
11. Arterial line (abbrev.)
15. Most common phlebotomy complication
16. Causes turbid serum
18. Stagnation of fluid
19. Relating to a vein
22. Saline _____ (VAD)
23. To search for a vein
26. Can cause an allergic reaction
28. Can be the result of nausea
32. Value can change 50% from A.M. to P.M.

Chapter Review Questions

1. The medical term for fainting is:
   a. edematous.
   b. exsanguination.
   c. reflux.
   d. syncope.

2. According to CAP guidelines, drugs that interfere with blood tests should be stopped:
   a. 1 to 4 hours before the test.
   b. 4 to 24 hours prior to the test.
   c. 24 to 48 hours prior to the test.
   d. 48 to 72 hours prior to the test.

3. Which of the following tests is affected the most if collected from a crying infant?
   a. Bilirubin
   b. Cholesterol
   c. Lead level
   d. WBC count

4. A hematoma may result from:
   a. inadequate site pressure applied after a venipuncture.
   b. needle penetration through the back wall of the vein.
   c. using a needle that is too large for the size of the vein.
   d. All of the above can result in hematoma formation.

5. Results of this test have a direct correlation with the patient's age.
   a. Blood culture
   b. Creatinine clearance
   c. Glucose
   d. Hemoglobin

6. Which of the following specimen conditions would lead you to suspect that the patient was not fasting when it was collected?
   a. Cloudy white serum
   b. Pale-yellow plasma
   c. Pink to reddish plasma
   d. Yellowish brown serum

7. A phlebotomist needs to collect a plasma specimen for a coagulation test. The patient has an IV in the left arm near the wrist and a hematoma in the antecubital area of the right arm. Which of the following is the best place to collect the specimen?
   a. Above the IV
   b. From the IV after shutting it off for 2 minutes
   c. Distal to the hematoma
   d. All of the above are acceptable collection sites

8. A patient's arm is in anatomical position. There appears to be a loop under the skin between the wrist and the elbow. You feel a buzzing sensation when you touch it. What you are most likely feeling is:
   a. an AV graft.
   b. an implanted port.
   c. a PICC.
   d. a sclerosed vein.

9. While you are in the middle of drawing a blood specimen, your patient starts to faint. The first thing you should do is:
   a. apply a cold compress directly to the patient's forehead.
   b. grab ammonia inhalant and wave it near the patient's nose.
   c. quickly release the tourniquet and remove the needle.
   d. tell the patient to lower the head and breathe deeply.

10. A patient has had a mastectomy on the left side and has an IV midway down the right arm. Where is the best place to perform a venipuncture?
    a. Above the IV on the right arm
    b. Below the IV on the right arm
    c. In the left antecubital area
    d. In the left hand or wrist

11. Blood loss to a point where life cannot be sustained is called:
    a. diurnal variation.
    b. exsanguination.
    c. iatrogenic anemia.
    d. vasovagal syncope.

12. Which of the following specimens would most likely be rejected for testing?
    a. A hemolyzed potassium specimen
    b. An icteric bilirubin specimen
    c. A nonfasting glucose specimen
    d. An underfilled serum tube

13. Which of the following is a clue that you have accidentally punctured an artery instead of a vein?
    a. The blood is dark bluish red.
    b. The blood spurts into the tube.
    c. The patient feels great pain.
    d. All of the above are clues.

14. The serum or plasma of a hemolyzed specimen would most likely look:
    - a. cloudy or turbid.
    - b. pale yellow.
    - c. pinkish to red.
    - d. yellowish brown.

15. Underfilling this tube will most likely result in a hemolyzed specimen.
    - a. EDTA tube
    - b. Light-blue top
    - c. Gray top
    - d. SST

16. Which activity can contaminate a blood specimen and affect the testing performed on it?
    - a. Cleaning the site with alcohol before drawing an ETOH specimen.
    - b. Collecting blood cultures before the povidone–iodine is totally dry.
    - c. Using povidone–iodine to clean the site prior to a finger puncture.
    - d. All of the above activities can affect testing done on the specimen.

17. Which activity is least likely to lead to failure to draw blood?
    - a. Choosing a vein that has patency
    - b. Leaving the tourniquet on too long
    - c. Loosely anchoring the vein
    - d. Using a tube that was dropped

18. The best way to keep a vein from rolling is to:
    - a. insert the needle at a 45-degree angle.
    - b. make certain to anchor it well.
    - c. tie the tourniquet very tight.
    - d. use a large-diameter needle.

19. You insert the needle in a patient's arm and properly engage the tube. No blood flows into the tube. You make subtle needle adjustments and there is still no blood flow. Which of the following is the best thing to do next?
    - a. Discontinue the draw and try somewhere else.
    - b. Keep redirecting the needle until you hit a vein.
    - c. Lift up on the needle to create a steeper angle.
    - d. Try a new tube in case it is a vacuum problem.

20. Which of the following is the most likely to affect test results?
    - a. Edema
    - b. Petechiae
    - c. Reflux
    - d. Syncope

Case Studies

Case Study 9-1: Problem Sites, Complications, and Procedural Errors

Erica is a recent phlebotomy program graduate who was hired less than a month ago by a major hospital in her first job as a phlebotomist. Her first 3 months of employment are a probationary period, and she is determined to do a good job. This morning she has been asked to collect a stat CBC and electrolytes from a patient in an intensive care unit. The patient is responsive and cooperative but has difficulty breathing. The patient's nurse mentions that she will hook up the patient's oxygen therapy as soon as the phlebotomist is finished with him. He has an IV in his left hand. Erica palpates the right antecubital area. She can feel the median cubital vein, but it is deep. The basilic vein is visible and prominent, so she decides to use it to collect the specimen. When she inserts the needle into the arm, the vein rolls and her needle ends up beside the vein and slightly under it. She redirects the needle and the vein rolls again. The patient winces in pain but says nothing. Noticing the look of pain on the patient's face, Erica asks him if it hurts. The patient says yes and tells her that the pain is radiating down his arm and his fingers are tingling. Erica asks him if he would like her to remove the needle. The patient replies "No,

you've got to get the specimen," so Erica tries again to redirect the needle. Finally, blood spurts into the tube and a hematoma starts to form quickly. At first Erica thinks that she may have hit an artery, but the specimen is normal in color, so Erica dismisses the thought. She quickly collects the specimens, covers the site with gauze, and asks the patient to hold pressure while she labels the tubes. When she has finished she thanks the patient and delivers the stat specimens to the laboratory.

QUESTIONS

1. What site selection issues were associated with the collection of this specimen?

2. Were the site selection issues handled properly? Explain why or why not.

3. What complications and procedural errors were involved?

4. Were complications and procedural errors handled properly? Explain why or why not.

Case Study 9-2: Specimen Quality Concerns

Ray, a newly hired phlebotomist who has just recently finished phlebotomy training, is preparing to draw the last GTT specimen on an outpatient. This is the first GTT he has performed without supervision, and he is proud of how well he has done. The patient has good veins in both arms, so he has been alternating arms for the blood draws. The patient is anxious to go home and Ray is in a hurry to go on break, so he quickly selects a vein, performs a successful venipuncture, and collects the required gray-top tube. He finishes the draw and quickly shakes the tube. Later, as he starts to label it, he notices that the tube is only half full. He has been allowed to submit other partial tubes without a problem, so he shrugs his shoulders and proceeds to bandage and then dismiss the patient. He submits the specimen to the laboratory and goes on break. When he returns he is informed that the last GTT specimen was

hemolyzed and unsuitable for testing, so that the test will have to be repeated. Ray is completely surprised by this because there were no problems with the draw. Now Ray has to call the patient and reschedule the test. The patient is understandably upset.

QUESTIONS

1. What errors did Ray make that could have caused hemolysis of the specimen?

2. What could Ray have done differently that might have prevented the hemolysis?

3. What other error did Ray make?

4. What could Ray have done differently to prevent the error in number 3 above?

Case Study 9-3: Damaged Tube

Phyllis had been doing outpatient phlebotomy for years, but for some reason that morning she wasn't her usual careful self. It was a very busy day. She was by herself and trying to work as fast as she could. She had already drawn 10 patients, but there were quite a few more still in the waiting area. Her eleventh patient was a young man who needed a specimen drawn for a bilirubin and GGT. As she reached above the draw station to grab the required gel tube and a spare out of the rack, one slipped through her fingers, bounced off the counter and landed on the floor. She quickly picked it up, wiped the top with an alcohol pad and proceeded with the draw. The man had great veins and she easily inserted the needle. To her surprise, the gel tube started to disintegrate as she pushed it into the holder and just as the blood started to flow into it. A piece of plastic that had one end stuck in the tube gel pierced her glove. She quickly pulled the broken tube out of the holder, inserted the spare, and continued the draw while the young man watched in astonishment. As the new tube filled she grabbed a tissue and wiped her glove, which was splashed with blood from the broken tube. Amazingly, although there was also blood on the counter and floor, none got on the patient.

She finished the draw, remarked how that had never happened before, bandaged the patient and sent him on his way. As she removed her gloves and washed her hands she discovered that the broken piece of tube had not only pierced her glove, it had also pierced her thumb. She cleaned her thumb, the counter, and the floor and went back to drawing patients. She filled out an incident report before she left at the end of the day. Several weeks later she noticed the whites of her eyes looked a bit yellow.

QUESTIONS

1. How could Phyllis have prevented this accident?

2. What could have caused the tube to disintegrate?

3. What is it called when the whites of the eyes look yellow, and what could have caused that to happen to Phyllis?

4. What information about this patient draw should have given her an idea that this specimen was a health hazard for her?

5. What employee health rule did she ignore?

Chapter 10

Capillary Puncture Equipment and Procedures

Objectives

Study the information in your TEXTBOOK that corresponds to each objective to prepare yourself for the activities in this chapter.

1 Define and use capillary puncture terminology, identify capillary puncture equipment, and list the order of draw for capillary specimens and describe the theory behind it.

2 Describe capillary specimen composition, identify differences between capillary, arterial, and venous specimen composition and reference values, decide when capillary puncture is indicated, and demonstrate knowledge of site selection criteria.

3 Describe how to collect capillary specimens from adults, infants, and children, describe specimen collection procedures and explain the clinical significance of capillary blood gas, neonatal bilirubin, and newborn screening tests, and name tests that cannot be performed on capillary specimens and explain why.

4 Describe how to prepare both routine and thick blood smears, give reasons why they are sometimes made at the collection site, and identify tests performed on them.

Matching

Use choices only once unless otherwise indicated.

MATCHING 10-1: KEY TERMS AND DESCRIPTIONS

Match each key term with the *best* description.

Key Terms (1–10)

1. _____ arterialized

2. _____ blood film/smear

3. _____ calcaneus

4. _____ CBGs

5. _____ cyanotic

6. _____ differential

7. _____ feather

8. _____ galactosemia

9. _____ hypothyroidism

10. _____ interstitial fluid

Descriptions

A. A drop of blood spread thin on a microscope slide
B. Bluish in color from lack of oxygen
C. Capillary blood gases; blood gas tests on a capillary specimen
D. Disorder characterized by an inherited inability to metabolize a milk sugar
E. Disorder characterized by insufficient levels of thyroid hormones
F. Fluid in the tissue spaces between the cells
G. Medical term for heel bone
H. Microscopic examination of a blood smear to identify number, type, and characteristics of blood cells
I. Term used to describe a capillary specimen collected from a warmed site
J. Thinnest area of a properly made blood smear where a differential is performed

Key Terms (11–20)

11. _____ intracellular fluid

12. _____ lancet

13. _____ microhematocrit tubes

14. _____ microtubes

15. _____ neonatal screening

16. _____ osteochondritis

17. _____ osteomyelitis

18. _____ PKU

19. _____ posterior curvature

20. _____ whorls

Descriptions

A. Back of the heel
B. Disorder involving a defect in the metabolism of phenylalanine
C. Fluid within the cells
D. Inflammation of the bone and cartilage
E. Inflammation of the bone marrow and adjacent bone
F. Narrow-bore 50 to 75 mL capillary tubes
G. Routine testing of newborns for the presence of certain disorders
H. Sharp-pointed or bladed instrument used for capillary puncture
I. Special small plastic tubes used to collect capillary specimens
J. Spiral pattern of the fingerprint

MATCHING 10-2: FINGER PUNCTURE PRECAUTION AND RATIONALE

Match the finger puncture precaution with the appropriate rationale.

Finger Puncture Precaution

1. _____ *Do not* puncture fingers of infants and children under 1 year of age.

2. _____ *Do not* puncture fingers on the same side as a mastectomy without permission from the patient's physician.

3. _____ *Do not* puncture parallel to the grooves or lines of the fingerprint.

Finger Puncture Rationale

A. A puncture in line with a fingerprint groove makes collection difficult because it allows blood to run down the finger rather than form a rounded drop that is easier to collect.
B. It has a pulse, indicating an artery in the puncture area, and the skin is generally thicker and more calloused, making it difficult to obtain a good specimen.
C. The amount of tissue between skin surface and bone is so small that bone injury is very likely. Known complications include infection and gangrene
D. The arm is susceptible to infection, and effects of lymphostasis can lead to erroneous results.

4. _____ *Do not* puncture the fifth or little (pinky) finger.

5. _____ *Do not* puncture the index finger.

6. _____ *Do not* puncture the side or very tip of the finger.

7. _____ *Do not* puncture the thumb.

E. The distance between the skin surface and bone is half as much at the side and tip as it is in the central fleshy portion of the finger.

F. It is usually more calloused and harder to puncture, more sensitive, so the puncture can be more painful, and it is typically used more, so a patient may notice the pain longer.

G. The tissue between the skin surface and bone is thinnest in this finger, and bone injury is likely.

MATCHING 10-3: HEEL PUNCTURE PRECAUTION AND RATIONALE

Heel Puncture Precaution

1. _____ *Do not* puncture any deeper than 2 mm.

2. _____ *Do not* puncture areas between the imaginary boundaries.

3. _____ *Do not* puncture bruised areas.

4. _____ *Do not* puncture in the arch and any areas of the foot other than the heel.

5. _____ *Do not* puncture sites that are swollen.

6. _____ *Do not* puncture the posterior curvature of the heel.

7. _____ *Do not* puncture through previous puncture sites.

Heel Puncture Rationale

A. Arteries, nerves, tendons, and cartilage in these areas can be injured.

B. Deeper punctures risk injuring the bone, even in the safest puncture areas.

C. Excess tissue fluid in the area could contaminate the specimen.

D. It can be painful and impaired circulation or byproducts of the healing process can negatively affect the specimen.

E. The bone can be as little as 1 mm deep in this area.

F. The calcaneus may be as little as 2 mm deep in this area.

G. This can be painful and can spread previously undetected infection.

MATCHING 10-4: BLOOD SMEAR PROBLEM AND PROBABLE CAUSE

Match the blood smear problem with a probable cause (TEXT Table 10-4). Use choices only once.

Problem

1. _____ Absence of feather

2. _____ Holes in smear

3. _____ Ridges or uneven thickness

4. _____ Smear is too thick

5. _____ Smear is too short

6. _____ Smear is too long

7. _____ Smear is too thin

8. _____ Streaks or tails in feathered edge

Probable Cause

A. Blood drop too small

B. Dirty slide or fat globules in the blood

C. Edge of spreader slide dirty or chipped

D. Spreader slide angle too shallow

E. Spreader slide lifted before smear was completed

F. Spreader slide pushed too quickly

G. Patient has high red blood cell count

H. Too much pressure applied to spreader slide

Labeling Exercises

LABELING EXERCISE 10-1: ADULT HAND

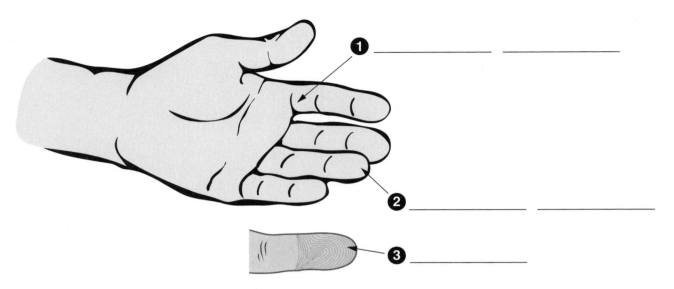

Use directional medical terminology to label the finger parts indicated by arrows 1 and 2. Place an "R" on the fingers that are recommended as capillary puncture sites. Place "NR" on the fingers that are not recommended as capillary puncture sites. Draw a red line to indicate the direction of puncture on an acceptable area of the finger segment identified by arrow number 3. Identify the term for the pattern of the fingerprint shown on the finger segment, and write it on the line after arrow number 3.

LABELING EXERCISE 10-2: INFANT FOOT

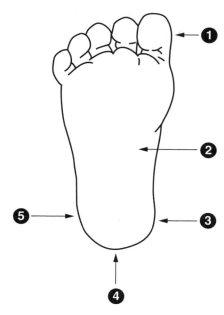

Identify the areas of the infant foot identified by the numbered arrows and write the term for the area on the corresponding numbered line. Use directional medical terms for numbers 3, 4, and 5. In parentheses after each term, write the letter "R" if the site is a recommended heel puncture site and the letters "NR" if it is not a recommended site for heel puncture. Draw dotted lines to indicate the imaginary lines that are used to determine the safe areas for heel puncture. Color the safe areas for heel puncture pink. Draw an "X" in the area of the heel bone and write the medical term for heel bone on line 6 below.

1. _____ 4. _____

2. _____ 5. _____

3. _____ 6. _____

Knowledge Drills

KNOWLEDGE DRILL 10-1: CAUTION AND KEY POINT RECOGNITION

The following sentences are from "CAUTION and KEY POINT" statements found throughout Chapter 10 in the TEXTBOOK. Using the TEXTBOOK, fill in the blanks with the missing information.

1. Sometimes (A) _____ blood obtained by (B) _____ during (C) _____ draw situations is put into (D) _____. When this is done, the specimen must be labeled as (E) _____ blood. Otherwise, it will be assumed to be a (F) _____ specimen, which may have different (G) _____ (H) _____.

2. Capillary puncture is generally *not* appropriate for patients who are (A) _____ or have poor (B) _____ to the (C) _____ from other causes, such as shock, because (D) _____ may be hard to obtain and may not be (E) _____ of (F) _____ elsewhere in the body.

3. The temperature of the material used to (A) _____ the (B) _____ must not exceed (C) _____ (_____) because higher temperatures can (D) _____ the skin, especially the delicate skin of an (E) _____.

4. *Do not* use (A) _____ (B) _____ to clean skin puncture sites because it greatly interferes with a number of tests, most notably bilirubin, (C) _____ acid, (D) _____, and (E) _____.

5. *Do not* squeeze, use strong (A) _____ pressure, or (B) "_____" the site, as (C) _____ and (D) _____ (E) _____ contamination of the specimen can result.

6. *Do not* use a (A) _____ motion against the (B) _____ of the skin and attempt to collect blood as it flows (C) _____ the (D) _____. (E) _____ the (F) _____ of the microtube against the skin activates (G) _____ causing them to (H) _____, and can also (I) _____ the specimen.

7. *Do not* apply (A) _____ to infants and children under (B)_____ years of age because they pose a (C) _____ hazard. In addition, bandage (D) _____ can (E) _____ to the paper-thin skin of newborns and (F) _____ it when the (G) _____ is removed.

8. The (A) _____ (B) _____ must be (C) _____ (D) _____ when collecting a bilirubin specimen to prevent it from breaking down the (E) _____ in the specimen as it is collected.

9. If an infant requires a (A) _____ (B)_____, newborn screening samples should be collected (C) _____ it is started, as (D) _____ of the sample with (E) _____ blood invalidates test results.

10. *Do not* contaminate the filter paper (A) _____ by touching them with or without (B) _____ or allowing any other object or substance to touch them before, during, or (C) _____ specimen collection. Substances that have been identified as (D) _____ in newborn screening specimens include (E) _____, formula, lotion, powder, and (F) _____.

11. Blood (A) _____ are considered (B) _____ or (C) _____

    material until they are (D) _____ or fixed.

12. Capillary specimen collection is especially useful for (A) _____ patients in whom removal of

    (B) _____ quantities of blood by venipuncture can have (C) _____ (D) _____.

13. An important (A) _____-required lancet safety feature is a permanently (B) _____

    blade or (C) _____ (D) _____ to reduce the risk of accidental sharps injury.

14. Although (A) _____ (B) _____ microtubes are available from some manufacturers,

    they are not to be used for (C) _____ specimens. They are intended to be used for

    (D) _____ (E) _____ collected by (F) _____ in difficult draw situations.

15. Pay strict attention to (A) _____ (B) _____ of microtubes containing (C) _____.

KNOWLEDGE DRILL 10-2: SCRAMBLED WORDS

Unscramble the following words using the hints given in parenthesis and the letters that have been placed in the correct boxes. Finish writing the correct spelling of the scrambled word in the corresponding boxes.

1. zalitraerdie (blood from a warmed site)

		t			i			i			

2. liribunbi (it can cross the blood–brain barrier)

	i			r			i	

3. slacneuca (do not puncture this)

	a		c		e		

4. placryail (this bed is in the skin)

		p			l		r	

5. snatrelititi (pertaining to spaces between tissue cells)

		t			s		i	t			

6. cletan (a very sharp object)

		n	c		

7. napartl (pertaining to the sole of the foot)

		a		t		

8. pocos (not good technique to do this)

			o	

9. tairoluvtel (light that breaks down bilirubin)

					V		O	L	r	

10. slowhr (fingerprint pattern)

	h				s

KNOWLEDGE DRILL 10-3: TRUE/FALSE ACTIVITY

The following statements are all false. Circle the one or two words that make the statement false and write the correct word/s that would make the statement true in the space provided.

1. Microhematocrit tubes are often referred to as "bullets" because of their size and shape.

2. Warming a capillary puncture site can increase blood flow up to 10 times.

3. Capillary puncture is sometimes recommended when available veins are fragile or must be saved for other procedures such as a glucose tolerance test.

4. Except for POCT methods, blood specimens for glucose tests cannot be collected by capillary puncture.

5. Microtubes for chemistry specimens are collected first in the order of draw for capillary puncture.

6. The CLSI recommended site for capillary puncture on adults and children older than 1 year is the palmar surface of the distal or end segment of the middle or ring finger of the dominant hand.

7. The safest area for heel puncture is the medial or lateral palmar surface of the heel.

8. Neonatal bilirubin specimens must be kept cool during transportation and handling.

9. Phenylketonuria is a temporarily acquired disorder.

10. Blood spot circles for newborn screening tests are filled by applying a large drop of free-flowing blood to each side of the filter paper.

Skills Drills

SKILLS DRILL 10-1: REQUISITION ACTIVITY

Any Hospital USA
1123 West Physician Drive
Any Town USA

Laboratory Test Requisition

- -

PATIENT INFORMATION:

Name: _____ Smith _____ John _____ L _____
                   (last)   (first)   (MI)

Identification Number: __051263975_____ Birth Date: _____

Referring Physician: __Payne_____

Date to be Collected: __05/12/2015_____ Time to be Collected: __STAT____

Special Instructions: __Collect by capillary puncture only_____

- -

TEST(S) REQUIRED:

_____ NH4 – Ammonia	_____ Gluc – glucose
__X__ Bili – Bilirubin, total & direct	_____ Hgb – hemoglobin
_____ BMP – basic metabolic panel	_____ Lact – lactic acid/lactate
_____ BUN – Blood urea nitrogen	_____ Plt. Ct. – platelet count
__X__ Lytes – electrolytes	_____ PT – prothrombin time
__X__ CBC – complete blood count	_____ PTT – partial thromboplastin time
_____ Chol – cholesterol	_____ RPR – rapid plasma reagin
_____ ESR – erythrocyte sed rate	_____ T&S – type and screen
_____ EtOH – alcohol	_____ PSA – prostate specific antigen
_____ D-dime	

You have received the following test order with instructions to collect the specimens by capillary puncture. List (according to the order of draw) the name of the test that will be collected in each tube, the stopper colors of the microtubes you will use, the additive(s) the tubes contain (if any), and any special handling required for each specimen. Write "NA" if no special handling is required.

Test in Order of Draw	Stopper Color	Tube Additive	Special Handling
1. _____	_____	_____	_____
2. _____	_____	_____	_____
3. _____	_____	_____	_____

SKILLS DRILL 10-2: WORD BUILDING

Divide each of the words below into all of its elements (parts); prefix (P), word root (WR), combining vowel (CV), and suffix (S). Write the word part and its definition on the corresponding lines. Write the general meaning of the word in the space provided. If the word does not have a particular element, write "NA" (not applicable) in its place. (See Chapter 4 of the TEXTBOOK.)

Example: Pathologist

Elements _____*NA*_____ / _____*path*_____ / _____*o*_____ / _____*logist*_____
                     P   WR   CV   S

Definitions _____*NA*_____ / _____*disease*_____ / _____*NA*_____ / _*specialist in the study of*_

Meaning: a specialist who studies and interprets disease

1. osteochondritis

Elements _____ / _____ / _____ / _____ / _____
               P   WR   CV   WR   S

Definitions _____ / _____ / _____ / _____ / _____

Meaning:

2. microhematocrit

Elements _____ / _____ / _____ / _____
               P   WR   CV   S

Definitions _____ / _____ / _____ / _____

Meaning:

3. hemolyze

Elements _____ / _____ / _____ / _____
               P   WR   CV   S

Definitions _____ / _____ / _____ / _____

Meaning:

4. hypothyroidism

Elements _____ / _____ / _____ / _____
               P   WR   CV   S

Definitions _____ / _____ / _____ / _____

Meaning:

5. dermal

Elements _____ / _____ / _____ / _____
               P   WR   CV   S

Definitions _____ / _____ / _____ / _____

Meaning:

6. cyanotic

Elements _____ / _____ / _____ / _____
               P   WR   CV   S

Definitions _____ / _____ / _____ / _____

Meaning:

7. neonatal

Elements _____ / _____ / _____ / _____
               P   WR   CV   S

Definitions _____ / _____ / _____ / _____

Meaning:

Chapter 10: Capillary Puncture Equipment and Procedures

SKILLS DRILL 10-3: FINGERSTICK PROCEDURE (Text Procedure 10-1)

Fill in the blanks with the missing information.

Steps

1 to 4. See Chapter 8 Venipuncture steps 1 through 4.

5. Position the patient.

6. Select the puncture site.

7. (5) _____ the site, if applicable.

8. Clean and (8) _____ the site.

9. Prepare equipment.

10. Grasp finger or heel firmly.

11. Position lancet, puncture site, and discard lancet.

Explanation/Rationale

See Chapter 8 Procedure 8-2: steps 1 through 4.

CLSI standards require the patient to be seated, or reclining in an appropriate chair, or lying down. The arm must be supported on a (1) _____ surface and the hand palm up. **Note:** A young child may have to be held on the lap and restrained by a parent or guardian.

Selecting an appropriate site protects the patient from (2)_____, allows collection of a (3) _____ specimen, and prevents spreading previous (4) _____.

(6)_____ the site makes blood collection easier and faster and reduces the tendency to (7) _____ the site. It is not normally part of a routine fingerstick unless the hand is cold, in which case, wrap it in a comfortably warm washcloth or towel for 3 to 5 minutes or use a commercial warming device.

Cleaning with (9) _____ (10)_____ alcohol removes or inhibits skin flora that could infiltrate the puncture and cause infection. Allowing the site to dry (11)_____ permits maximum (12) _____ action, prevents contamination caused by wiping, and avoids stinging on puncture and specimen (13) _____ from residual alcohol.

Selecting and preparing equipment in advance of use helps ensure that the correct equipment is ready and within reach for the procedure. (14) _____ opening packaging aids in infection control.

Grasping the finger or heel firmly prevents sudden movement by the patient.

Holding the lancet between the thumb and index fingers of your (15) _____ hand (or as described by the device manufacturer) is required preparation for the puncture. Placing the lancet flat against the skin ensures good contact for the puncture. Discarding the lancet in sharps container (16) _____ after the puncture is a safety requirement that protects the patient, phlebotomist, and others from accidental injury or (17) _____ from the lancet.

12. Lower finger or heel and apply gentle (18) _____ until a blood drop forms

Lowering the appendage helps blood begin to flow (19)_____. Gentle pressure encourages blood flow without compromising specimen (20) _____.

13. Wipe away the (21) _____ blood drop.

Prevents contamination of the specimen with excess (22) _____ fluid and removes alcohol residue that could prevent formation of (23) _____ - _____ drops and also hemolyze the specimen.

14. Fill and (24) _____ the tubes/containers in order of draw.

(25) _____ tubes immediately after they are filled is necessary for proper (26) _____ function and to prevent (27) _____ in anticoagulant tubes. Following the order of draw for capillary specimens minimizes (28) _____ effects of clotting on specimens.

15. Place gauze, (29) _____ site, and apply pressure.

Absorbs excess blood, and helps stop (30) _____.

16. (31) _____ specimens and observe special (32) _____ instructions.

Prompt (33) _____ (see Chapter 8) helps ensure correct specimen (34) _____. Appropriate handling protects specimen (35) _____.

17. (36) _____ site and apply bandage.

Note: Do not apply a bandage to an infant or toddler.

Necessary to verify that bleeding has stopped. Bandaging keeps the site clean while the site (37) _____.

Note: If bleeding persists beyond (38) _____ notify the patient's physician or designated healthcare provider.

18. Dispose of used and (39) _____ materials.

Equipment packaging and bandage wrappers must be discarded in the trash. Follow (40) _____ protocol for discarding contaminated items, such as (41) _____ gauze.

19. Thank patient, parent, or guardian, remove and discard gloves, and (42) _____ hands.

Thanking the patient, parent or guardian is courteous and professional. Removing gloves (43) _____ and washing or decontaminating hands with (44) _____ is an infection control precaution.

20. Transport specimen to the lab.

(45) _____ delivery to the lab is necessary to protect specimen integrity.

SKILLS DRILL 10-4: HEELSTICK PROCEDURE RATIONALE (Text Procedure 10-2)

Match the rationale summary from the following list with the heelstick procedure steps listed below by placing the appropriate letter next to the step under Rationale Summary.

A. Absorbs excess blood and helps stop bleeding
B. An acceptable one is on the medial or lateral plantar surface of the heel
C. Doing this in advance helps ensure everything is ready and within reach
D. Encourages blood flow without compromising specimen integrity
E. Exposure to this can trigger a life-threatening reaction in some individuals
F. Follow facility protocol before doing this
G. Helps ensure correct specimen identification
H. Helps prevent sudden unexpected movement by the patient
I. Makes collection easier and reduces a tendency to squeeze the site
J. Must be reviewed for completeness
K. Necessary for proper additive function
L. Necessary to protect specimen integrity
M. Necessary to verify bleeding has stopped
N. Placing it flat against the skin ensures good contact for the puncture
O. Plays a major role in infection control
P. Prevents contamination of the specimen with excess tissue fluid
Q. Removes or inhibits skin flora that could cause infection
R. The infant should be lying face up with the foot lower than the torso
S. This is courteous and professional
T. Vital to patient safety and meaningful test results

Heelstick Procedure Step	**Rationale Summary**
1. Review and accession test request.	_____
2. Approach, identify, and prepare patient.	_____
3. Verify diet restrictions and latex sensitivity.	_____
4. Sanitize hands and put on gloves.	_____
5. Position the patient.	_____
6. Select the puncture site.	_____
7. Warm the site.	_____
8. Clean and air-dry the site.	_____
9. Prepare the equipment.	_____
10. Grasp the Heel Firmly	_____
11. Position lancet, puncture site, and discard lancet.	_____
12. Lower heel and apply gentle pressure until a blood drop forms	_____
13. Wipe away the first blood drop.	_____
14. Fill and mix tubes/containers in order of draw.	_____
15. Place gauze, elevate heel, and apply pressure.	_____
16. Label the specimen and observe special handling instructions.	_____
17. Check the site	_____
18. Dispose of used and contaminated materials	_____
19. Thank patient, parent or guardian, remove gloves, and sanitize hands.	_____
20. Transport specimen to the lab promptly.	_____

SKILLS DRILL 10-5: BLOOD SPOT COLLECTION PROCEDURE HIGHLIGHTS
(Text Procedure 10-4)

The following are highlights from the newborn screening blood spot collection procedure. Fill in the blanks with the missing information.

1. Bring the filter paper close to the heel: The (A) _____ must not actually (B) _____

   the (C) _____; if it does, (D) _____, incomplete (E) _____ of the paper,

   (F) _____, and stoppage of (G) _____ (H) _____can result.

2. Generate a large, free-flowing drop of blood: Small drops can result in incomplete (A) _____ and the

   tendency to (B) _____ successive drops in a circle to (C) _____ it.

3. Touch the blood drop to the center of the filter paper circle: The drop must touch the center of the circle for

   (A) _____ to (B) _____ (C) _____ out to the (D) _____.

4. Fill the circle with blood: Blood drop position must be (A) _____ until blood (B) _____

   through the circle, completely filling (C) _____ (D) _____ of the paper. Caution: Do not fill

   spots from the (E) _____ side to finish filling the circles because this causes (F) _____

   and (G) _____ test results.

5. Fill remaining blood spot circles: Fill (A) _____ circles the same way. (B) _____ or

   (C) _____ filled circles can result in (D) _____ to perform all required (E) _____.

6. Check the site: Examining the site is necessary to verify that bleeding has (A) _____. *Do not* apply

   a (B) _____ as it can become a (C) _____ hazard and can also (D) _____ the

   skin when removed.

7. Allow the specimen to air-dry: Air-drying in an elevated (A) _____ position

   away from heat or (B) _____is required for newborn screening specimens. They must not be

   (C) _____ to dry or (D) _____ with other specimens before, during, or after the

   drying process. (E) _____ or storage at a slant causes blood to (F) _____ to the

   (G) _____ end of the filter paper and leads to erroneous test results.

Crossword

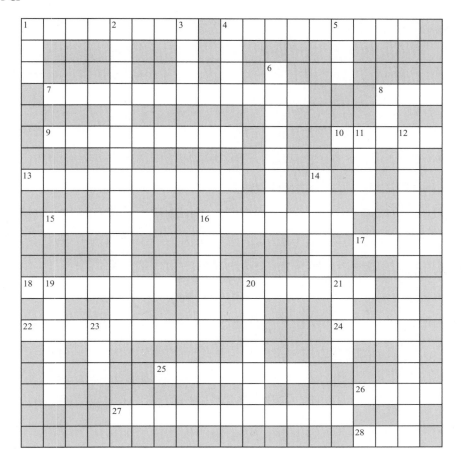

ACROSS

1. Marked by bluish color
4. Blood specimen type collected by a dermal puncture
7. Capillary blood becomes this after warming the site
8. Alcohol _____ used for cleaning the site
9. Heel bone
10. Digit not suggested for capillary collection
13. Small plastic tubes used to collect tiny amounts of blood
15. Rectangular glass plate required for making a blood smear
16. Clay for plugging microhematocrit tube
17. Testing done at the location of the patient (abbrev.)
18. Bottom surface of the foot
20. Spiral pattern of the fingerprint
22. Cuts in the skin
24. Place chosen to collect blood sample
25. Neonatal
26. Outer covering of the body
27. Contaminating factor when doing capillary collections (two words)
28. Hemolysis in newborns (abbrev.)

DOWN

1. Capillary blood gas (abbrev.)
2. Inflammation of the bone and cartilage
3. Regulations that establish standards for all laboratory facilities
4. Organization that offers phlebotomy standards
5. Leukocyte alkaline phosphatase
6. Pertaining to newborn
8. Genetic disorder associated with phenylalanine
11. Recommended collection site for infants
12. Term for obtaining tiny amounts of blood by capillary puncture
14. Recommended site for capillary puncture on children over 1 year of age
16. Container for used lancets and needles
19. Sterile, disposable, bladed instrument
20. Necessary to _____ first drop of blood
21. In order of draw, red-cap microtainer is collected _____
23. Units in the nursery where severely ill newborns can be monitored

Chapter Review Questions

1. An inherited metabolic disorder detected through newborn screening.
   a. Diabetes
   b. Glucose
   c. Phenylketonuria
   d. Potassium

2. Which of the following equipment is needed for a malaria test?
   a. Capillary tube
   b. Clay sealant
   c. Glass slide
   d. Microhematocrit tube

3. A plasma specimen for this type of test cannot be collected by capillary puncture.
   a. Chemistry
   b. Coagulation
   c. Hematology
   d. All of the above

4. Capillary blood composition more closely resembles
   a. arterial blood.
   b. lymph fluid.
   c. tissue fluid.
   d. venous blood.

5. The concentration of this analyte is normally lower in capillary specimens than in venous specimens
   a. calcium.
   b. glucose.
   c. hemoglobin.
   d. all of the above.

6. Capillary collection is the preferred method of blood collection in infants because
   a. an infant can be injured by the restraining method used.
   b. removing larger quantities of blood can lead to anemia.
   c. venipuncture may damage veins and surrounding tissue.
   d. all of the above.

7. If using capillary puncture to collect the following microtubes from a patient, which one would be collected first?
   a. Gray top
   b. Green top
   c. Purple top
   d. Red top

8. Which of the following is a recommended site for finger puncture in adults?
   a. End segment of the little finger
   b. Distal segment of the middle finger
   c. Plantar surface of the index finger
   d. Proximal segment of the ring finger

9. The medial plantar surface of the heel is located
   a. at the very back portion of the heel.
   b. in the middle of the bottom of the heel.
   c. on the big toe side of the bottom of the heel.
   d. on the little toe side of the bottom of the heel.

10. It is necessary to control the depth of lancet insertion during heel puncture to avoid
    a. bacterial contamination.
    b. bone injury.
    c. excessive bleeding.
    d. puncturing a vein.

11. The primary purpose of warming a capillary puncture site is to
    a. delay clotting.
    b. increase blood flow.
    c. minimize contamination.
    d. reduce hemoconcentration.

12. Skin pain fibers increase in abundance
    a. in the upper epidermis.
    b. below 2.4 mm in depth.
    c. beyond 4.9 mm in depth.
    d. within the vascular bed.

13. Adult capillary puncture may be performed when
    a. there are no accessible veins.
    b. the patient has thrombotic tendencies.
    c. veins must be saved for chemotherapy.
    d. all of the above.

14. Wipe away the first drop of blood during capillary puncture to
    a. minimize tissue fluid contamination
    b. reduce the chance of hemolysis.
    c. remove any alcohol residue.
    d. all of the above.

15. Do *not* use povidone–iodine to clean skin puncture sites because it interferes with
    a. potassium results.
    b. phosphorus results.
    c. uric acid results.
    d. all of the above.

16. Which of the following represents proper capillary specimen collection technique?
    a. Clean the site with alcohol and wipe it dry, so it will not sting.
    b. Puncture the skin parallel to the whorls of the fingerprint.
    c. Squeeze the finger hard to get the very best blood flow.
    d. Touch the scoop to the blood drop, not the skin surface.

17. Blood smears made using EDTA specimens should be prepared within
    a. 1 hour of specimen collection.
    b. 2 hours of specimen collection.
    c. 6 hours of specimen collection.
    d. 24 hours of specimen collection.

18. An infant bilirubin specimen is collected in an amber microtube to
    a. flag it as a capillary specimen.
    b. identify it as a bilirubin specimen.
    c. protect the specimen from light.
    d. reduce the chance of hemolysis.

19. Which of the following PKU collection techniques is incorrect?
    a. Air-dry the slips horizontally.
    b. Completely fill every circle.
    c. Do not touch the filter paper.
    d. Fill circles from both sides.

20. Which of the following can result in a blood smear that is too long?
    a. Angle of spreader slide is too steep.
    b. Blood drop is too large or too thin.
    c. Spreader slide is pushed too quickly.
    d. Patient has a high hemoglobin level.

Case Studies

Case Study 10-1: Neonatal Bilirubin Collection

A newly OJT (on the job) trained phlebotomist was sent to the newborn nursery to collect a bilirubin specimen. This was the first time she had collected an infant specimen by herself, and she was anxious to do a good job. The infant was under a UV light, and, although she thought it should be turned off, both nurses in the room were busy with a procedure on another infant and she didn't want to interrupt them to ask permission, so she decided to obtain the specimen quickly without turning it off. She rapidly cleaned the site and made the puncture. The blood came slowly and it took her a while to collect the specimen. She finally filled an amber bullet to an acceptable level, labeled it, put an adhesive bandage on the infant's heel, and delivered the specimen to the lab.

QUESTIONS

1. Why was the infant placed under a UV light?

2. Should the light have been turned off during specimen collection? Why or why not?

3. What might be the consequences of leaving the UV light on during specimen collection?

4. What could the phlebotomist have done to make the collection go more quickly?

5. What other error did the phlebotomist make that could have caused injury to the infant after she left the nursery?

Case Study 10-2: Capillary Specimen Collection Technique and Order of Draw

A phlebotomist had a request to collect STAT electrolytes on a patient and a CBC that was not STAT. The patient had an IV just above the wrist in the left arm. The right antecubital area was badly bruised, and the patient did not have any suitable veins in either hand. Consequently, the phlebotomist decided to collect the specimens by capillary puncture, choosing the right middle finger as the collection site. After making the puncture, the phlebotomist decided to collect the electrolytes first because they were STAT and he was having a difficult time getting good blood flow. He was able to fill the green top bullet for the electrolytes and proceeded to collect the CBC. He had to use a lot of pressure on the finger to keep the blood flowing, but he eventually filled a lavender bullet for the CBC to a proper level. After the samples had been submitted to the lab he was told to recollect the CBC because the results were questionable.

QUESTIONS

1. What was most likely wrong with the CBC results?

2. Why was only the CBC affected?

3. What could the phlebotomist have done differently to protect the CBC?

4. What should the phlebotomist do differently when he recollects the specimen?

Case Study 10-3: Newborn Screening Specimen Collection

Judy is a seasoned phlebotomist who has recently changed employers and now works in a busy women's hospital where lots of babies are born and lots of newborn screening specimens are collected. Judy has never really liked collecting newborn screening specimens and tries to avoid being the one who collects them. Today the phlebotomist who usually collects them is out sick, so Judy is given the assignment. Her first patient starts screaming at the top of his little lungs the minute she touches him. Just as she triggers the lancet blade he kicks really hard for a little guy and the lancet slips off heel. Only one side of the blade made contact with the heel. Blood does start to flow, but very slowly. She fills the first circle but has to use a lot of pressure to keep the blood flowing to fill the second one. She is finally able to fill the circles most of the way, but when she turns the filter paper over she sees that the blood did not soak all the way

through. By now the blood has stopped coming, so she grabs a new lancet and pokes the site again. This time the blood comes quickly and she is able to finish filling the circles from the back side of the form. It is time for her break, so she heads back to the lab with the form. She sets the form on its side on the counter and leaves it to dry while she heads off on her break.

QUESTIONS

1. Why do you think the blood came so slowly with the first puncture?

2. Identify three things that Judy did incorrectly while collecting the specimen.

3. She also handled the specimen improperly after collection. What did she do wrong and what effect could it have on the specimen?

Unit III Crossword Exercise

ACROSS

1. Antiseptics inhibit their growth
4. Spiral pattern that forms the fingerprint
6. Blood gas performed on ND (abbrev.)
8. Eutectic mixture of local anesthetics
9. Term used to describe milky white or turbid serum or plasma
11. Intravenous (abbrev.)
12. Anticoagulant typically used for hematology studies
13. Holding a vein in place by pulling the skin taut
15. Preanalytical errors can affect _____ results
16. Metabolism of glucose by blood cells
18. Record in the order received
20. ETS additive for blood culture specimens
22. Number that relates to the diameter of the needle lumen
23. Anticoagulant in tubes with light blue tops
25. Atrioventricular valve (abbrev.)
26. Property of thixotropic gel that changes during centrifugation
29. Pertaining to veins
30. Central venous access device
33. Excessive and persistent fear
37. Medical term for fainting
38. Examine by touch or feel

DOWN

1. Winged infusion set
2. Anticoagulants prevent it
3. Backflow of blood from an evacuated tube into a patient's vein
4. Do this to the site to arterialize a specimen
5. Internal space of a vessel or tube
7. Later product of red blood cell breakdown
10. Tiny red spots that appear on the skin upon tourniquet application
13. Substance that keeps blood from clotting
14. Destruction of RBCs and release of hemoglobin into the fluid of a specimen
17. Hardened
18. Prefix meaning against
19. Immediately
21. Container used to dispose of used needles and lancets
24. Condition characterized by high bilirubin levels
27. Combining form meaning bone
28. Fossa on ventral side of the arm (abbrev.)
31. Type of blood sampling device
32. Bedside or alternate site testing (abbrev.)
34. NB screening test for an amino acid metabolic disorder (abbrev.)
35. Written and signed order not to resuscitate (abbrev.)
36. Glass tube top color indicating no additive

Chapter 11

Special Collections and Point-of-Care Testing

Objectives

Study the information in your TEXTBOOK that corresponds to each objective to prepare yourself for the activities in this chapter.

1 Demonstrate basic knowledge of special collection procedures, define the associated terminology, and understand importance for special labeling, equipment, collection, timing and handling of each procedure.

2 Describe patient identification and specimen labeling procedures required for blood bank tests and identify the types of specimens typically required.

3 Describe sterile technique in blood culture collection, explain why it is important, and list the reasons why a physician might order blood cultures.

4 Define point-of-care testing (POCT), explain the principle behind the POCT examples listed in this chapter, and identify any special equipment required.

Matching

Use choices only once unless otherwise indicated.

MATCHING 11-1: KEY TERMS AND DESCRIPTIONS

Match the key term with the *best* description.

Key Terms (1–18)

1. _____ AABB
2. _____ ACT
3. _____ Aerobic
4. _____ Anaerobic
5. _____ ARD
6. _____ autologous
7. _____ BAC
8. _____ Bacteremia
9. _____ BNP
10. _____ Chain of custody
11. _____ Compatibility
12. _____ CRP
13. _____ EQC
14. _____ ETOH
15. _____ FAN
16. _____ FUO
17. _____ GTT
18. _____ HCG

Descriptions

A. Abbreviation for ethanol
B. Ability to be favorably mixed together
C. Activated clotting time
D. Antimicrobial removal device
E. Bacteria in the blood
F. Blood alcohol concentration
G. Donating blood for one's own use.
H. Fastidious antimicrobial neutralization
I. Fever of unknown origin
J. Hormone detected in pregnancy test
K. Instrument's electronic QC check
L. Measurement for congestive heart failure
M. Nonspecific marker for inflammation
N. Organization that sets guidelines for Blood Donor Centers
O. Special protocol for forensic specimen collections
P. Test to diagnose carbohydrate metabolism problems
Q. With air
R. Without air

Key Terms (19–37)

19. _____ Hypoglycemia
20. _____ Hyperkalemia
21. _____ Hypernatremia
22. _____ iCa2+
23. _____ INR
24. _____ K+
25. _____ Lactate
26. _____ Lookback
27. _____ Lysis
28. _____ NIDA
29. _____ Peak level
30. _____ POCT

Descriptions

A. After a meal
B. Decreased blood sugar levels
C. Heart muscle protein elevated in 3 to 6 hours
D. Heart muscle protein that may be elevated 14 days
E. Highest serum drug concentration anticipated
F. Increased blood potassium levels
G. Increased blood sodium levels
H. Intensive insulin therapy for glucose control
I. Ionized form of calcium
J. Lowest serum drug concentration expected
K. Microorganism and toxins in the blood
L. National Institute on Drug Abuse
M. Program to trace blood unit components to donor
N. Rupturing, as in the bursting of a red blood cell
O. Standardized form of PT results
P. Testing performed at the patient's side

31. _____ PP

32. _____ Septicemia

33. _____ TDM

34. _____ TGC

35. _____ TnI

36. _____ TnT

37. _____ Trough level

Q. The mineral potassium
R. Therapeutic drug levels collected at specific times
S. This analyte level marks severity of metabolic acidosis

MATCHING 11-2: POC TESTS AND INSTRUMENTS USED FOR TESTING

Match the following tests to the POCT instruments (instruments can only be used once).

POC Tests

A. CK-MB
B. Lactate
C. Glycosylated Hb
D. Hemoglobin
E. P_{CO_2}
F. PT
G. TnT
H. BUN
I. CRP
J. Hematocrit
K. β-ketone
L. UA
M. Guaiac
N. HCG
O. LDL
P. Platelet function

POCT Instruments

1. _____ Verify Now

2. _____ Quidel Quick Vue

3. _____ Precision XceedPro

4. _____ StatSpin CritSpin

5. _____ Hemoccult II Sensa

6. _____ CARDIAC T Rapid Assay

7. _____ Cholestech LDX

8. _____ Stratus CS

9. _____ GEM Premier 4000

10. _____ HemoCue HB 201+

11. _____ DCA Vantage

12. _____ Triage Cardiac Panel

13. _____ CoaguChek XS

14. _____ i-STAT

15. _____ ABL80

16. _____ Clinitek Advantus

MATCHING 11-3: SPECIAL TEST COLLECTION, EQUIPMENT, OR PROCEDURE

Match the following tests with the special equipment or procedure involved. (Answers can be used only once.)

Special Test

1. _____ 2-hour PP

2. _____ Blood alcohol

3. _____ Blood culture

4. _____ Blood type and screen

5. _____ RNA

6. _____ GTT

7. _____ Paternity testing

Special Handling, Equipment, or Procedure

A. Draw in trace element–free tube.
B. Involves intradermal injection of diluted antigen.
C. May require a proctor present at the time of collection.
D. May require photo identification before collection.
E. Requires serial collection of blood specimens at specific times.
F. Patient ID procedures are extra strict.
G. Requires a 9-to-1 ratio of blood to anticoagulant in the collection tube.
H. Skin antisepsis is critical to accurate test results.
I. Special chain of custody protocol required.

8. _____ Polycythemia

9. _____ PT

10. _____ TB test

11. _____ Urine drug screen

12. _____ Zinc

J. Specimen is collected at specific time after eating.
K. Treatment often involves removal of units of blood.
L. If not tested immediately, must be collected with a stabilizing reagent.

Labeling Exercises

LABELING EXERCISE 11-1: POC INSTRUMENTS AND TESTS

Label the photo of each of the following POC instruments with the name of the instrument and the test that it is used to measure. Choose from the following list of tests.

Instrument That Can Measure

ACT
b-ketones
Blood gases
BNP
Creatinine
HbA1c
hCG
HDL
Hematocrit
Hemoglobin
Lactate
Platelet function

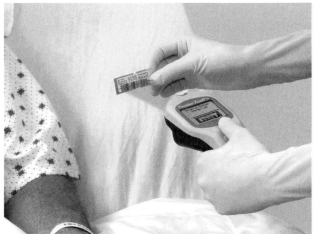

1. name: _____   test: _____

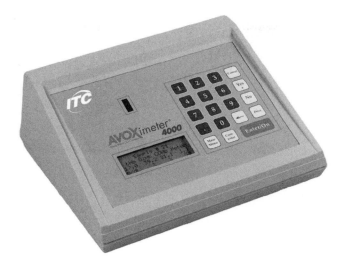

2. name: _____ test: _____

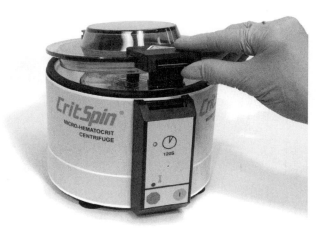

3. name: _____ test: _____

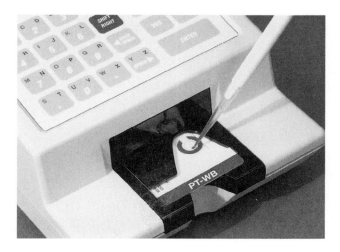

4. name: _____ test: _____

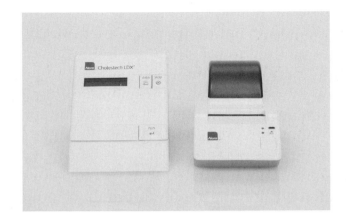

5. name: _____   test: _____

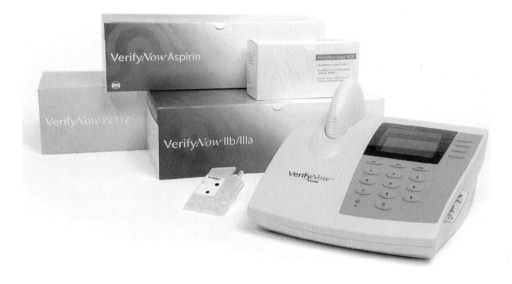

6. name: _____   test: _____

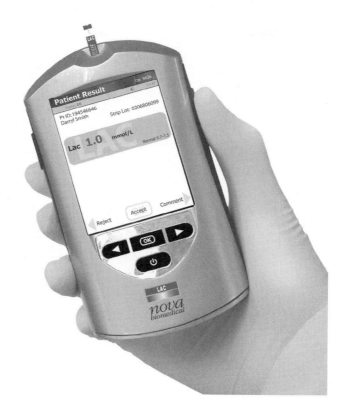

7. name: _____   test: _____

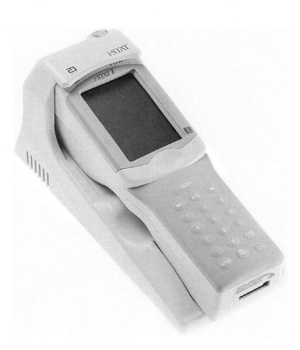

8. name: _____   test: _____

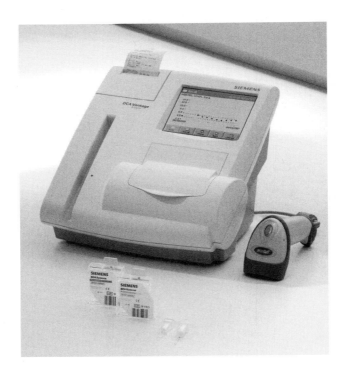

9. name: _____ test: _____

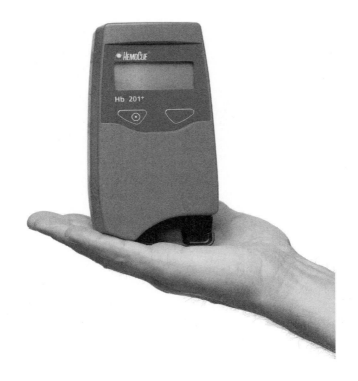

10. name: _____ test: _____

LABELING EXERCISE 11-2: ONE BBID SYSTEM

You are a new phlebotomist who is asked to get blood from a patient for a crossmatch STAT. Before leaving the laboratory with the requisition, the MT in the blood bank gives you a FlexiBlood form and band to use in collecting the specimen. When you get to the floor, you realize that you have several questions on how to use this form. Fortunately, adequate instructions for you to follow are given on the front of the form.

1. Which of the following is the unique BBID number? _____

2. Where does the preprinted patient information go? _____

3. Which part is filled in, removed, and placed on the band? _____

4. Which one is the label for the specimen tube? _____

5. What bar-code labels are to be put on the units in the laboratory? _____

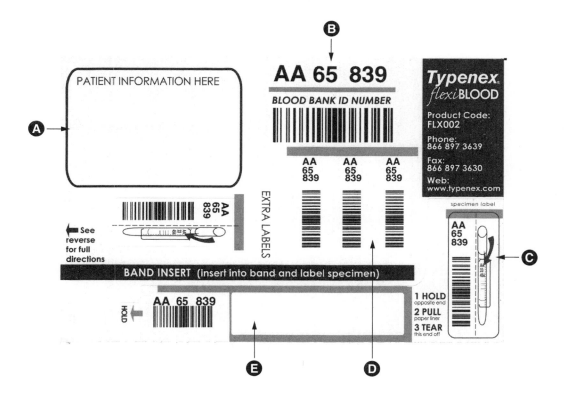

Knowledge Drills

KNOWLEDGE DRILL 11-1: CAUTION AND KEY POINT RECOGNITION

Instructions: The following sentences are taken from caution and key point statements found throughout the chapter. Using the TEXTBOOK, fill in the blanks with the missing information.

1. Blood cultures are typically ordered immediately (A) _____ or (B) _____

   (C) _____ spikes when bacteria are most likely to be present. (D) _____ collection is

   important, but (E) _____ is more important than (F) _____ in detecting the causative

   agent of septicemia.

2. When a (A) _____ is used to collect the blood, the (B) _____ bottle is filled first. When

   a (C) _____ is used, it is preferable to fill the (D) _____ bottle first because

   (E) _____ in the tubing will be drawn into it along with the blood.

3. According to the CLSI, (A) _____ (B) _____ is the recommended blood

   culture site disinfectant for (C) _____ 2 months and older and patients with (D) _____

   sensitivity.

4. Blood culture specimens are always collected (A) _____ in the order of draw to prevent

   (B) _____ from other (C) _____.

5. The practice of changing (A) _____ prior to this transferring blood from a syringe is no longer

   (B) _____. Several recent studies have shown that (C) _____ needles has little

   (D) _____ on reducing (E) _____ rates and may actually (F) _____

   risk of (G) _____ injury to the phlebotomist.

6. If the patient (A) _____ during the GTT procedure, his or her (B) _____ must be

   consulted to determine if the test should be (C) _____.

7. _____ tubes are preferred for blood alcohol specimens because of the (B) _____ nature

   of (C) _____ tubes.

8. Regulatory (A) _____ and the (B) _____ recommend that a person receive

   (C) _____ authorization to perform (D) _____ glucose testing only after

   completing (E) _____ training in facility-established procedures, including (F) _____ and

   (G) _____.

9. _____ should be repeated if the analyzer is (B) _____, the battery is

   (C) _____ or patient results or analyzer functioning are (D) _____.

10. A (A) _____ (B) _____ is also called a (C) _____ test after the purified

    (D) _____ derivative used in the test.

11. All (A) _____ tubes must be (B) _____ inverted (C) _____ to

    (D) _____ times immediately after collection to avoid (E) _____, which can

    (F) _____ test results.

12. When blood cultures from patients on (A) _____ therapy are ordered, they should be collected

    when the (B) _____ or other such drugs are at their (C) _____ concentration.

KNOWLEDGE DRILL 11-2: SCRAMBLED WORDS

Unscramble the following words using the hints given in parenthesis and the letters that have been placed in the correct boxes. Finish writing the correct spelling of the scrambled word in the corresponding box.

1. ampicestie (microbes in the bloodstream)

			t			e		i	

2. arcle (throw this tube away)

	l			

3. ayetprint (test to identify a father)

		t		r				

4. ceatiherput (beneficial)

	h			a		e				

5. eclotrane (capacity to endure without ill effects)

			e				e	

6. gloxticooy (the study of poisons)

			i			o		

7. guloosotau (donor and recipient are the same)

	u			l				s	

8. laedslogycyt (sugar chemically linked to protein)

		y		s				t		

9. ralispopdant (after eating)

			t		r				a	

10. spitansesi (prevention of infection by inhibiting microbes)

			i	s				s	

KNOWLEDGE DRILL 11-3: TRUE/FALSE

The following statements are all false. Circle the one or two words that make the statement false and write the correct word(s) that would make the statement true in the space provided.

1. Blood bank tests require the collection of one or more gray or pink top EDTA tubes.

2. For FUO, two to three cultures should be collected, one right after another from the same sites.

3. The same methods for blood culture skin antisepsis for adults apply to pediatric patients unless the antiseptic is Chloroprep.

4. To minimize the risk of contamination by skin flora, the collection sites require a 15 to 20 second friction scrub to get to the bacteria beneath the dead skin cells onto the surface of the arm.

5. When a test for lead is ordered, the blood specimen must be sent for testing immediately or collected in a special stabilizing reagent.

6. When a trace element test is ordered, it is best to draw it last if using a needle/tube assembly.

7. Coagulation specimens drawn through VADs require a discard volume of blood that is ten times the dead-space volume of the tubing, approximately 5 mL.

8. A GTT patient is not allowed to drink water or chew gum, as these activities stimulate the digestive process and may cause erroneous test results.

9. Urine samples are preferred for paternity testing; however, buccal swabs are increasingly being used.

10. Drug screening tests are typically performed on saliva rather than blood because it is easy to obtain and a wide variety of drugs or their metabolites can be detected in urine for a longer period of time.

KNOWLEDGE DRILL 11-4: GLUCOSE TOLERANCE TEST (GTT)

Background: A glucose tolerance test (GTT) is used to diagnose carbohydrate metabolism problems. The major carbohydrate in the blood is glucose, the body's source of energy. The hormone insulin, produced by the pancreas, is primarily responsible for regulating blood glucose levels. The GTT evaluates insulin response to a measured dose of glucose by recording glucose levels on specimens collected at specific time intervals. Results are plotted on a graph, creating what is referred to a GTT curve.

Instructions: The fasting blood glucose for a GTT was collected from a patient at 05:00 hours. The blood was tested and the value was normal. The patient was given the glucose drink at 05:25 hours and finished drinking it at 05:30 hours.

1. Fill in the rest of the GTT collection times in the table below.

2. Using the collection times and the results below, graph the glucose absorption curve.

3. Based on Figure 11–12 and GTT curves in Chapter 11, check which of the following is correct: This graph is

   _____ normal or _____ abnormal.

Timing of GTT	Collection Time	Results
Fasting	05:00	75 mg/dL
0.5 hour		250 mg/dL
1.0 hour		200 mg/dL
2.0 hours		175 mg/dL
3.0 hours		150 mg/dL

KNOWLEDGE DRILL 11-5: EXAMPLES OF DRUGS NEEDING THERAPEUTIC MONITORING AND THEIR USE

Instructions: Match each DRUG CATEGORY in the middle column below with an EXAMPLE and USE by drawing an arrow between the columns to the appropriate answer. Use a different-colored pen or pencil for each arrow. Answers can be used only once.

Drug Example	Drug Category	Drug Usage
Amikacin	Bronchodilators	Epilepsy
Methotrexate	Protease inhibitors	Bipolar disorder
Tegretol	Chemotherapy drugs	Asthma
Doxepin	Psychiatric drugs	Psoriasis
Theophylline	Antibiotics and Antifungals	Autoimmune disorders
Digitoxin	Cardiac drugs	Angina
Cyclosporine	Anticonvulsants	HIV/AIDS
Atazanavir	Immunosuppressants	Resistant infections

Skills Drills

SKILLS DRILL 11-1: REQUISITION ACTIVITY

Instructions: Answer the following questions concerning the test requisition shown below.

1. How many BC media bottles will be needed to complete this order? _____

_____

2. If the physician wants these blood cultures performed as quickly as possible, how many BCs can be drawn at the same time and from where? _____

_____

3. Describe the special collection technique that must be used before obtaining these samples. _____

_____

4. To be more efficient, should the phlebotomist ask the nurse to collect it from the heparin lock that is in the right forearm? Explain. _____

_____

Any Hospital USA
1123 West Physician Drive
Any Town USA

Laboratory Test Requisition

- -

PATIENT INFORMATION:

Name: _____ Smith _____ George _____ L _____
　　　　　　　(last)　　　　(first)　　　　(MI)

Identification Number: __09365784__　　　Birth Date: __06/21/75__

Referring Physician: __Hurstmatson__

Date to be Collected: __05/20/15__　　　Time to be Collected: __STAT__

Special Instructions: __need to start antibiotics ASAP__

- -

TEST(S) REQUIRED:

_____ NH4 – Ammonia	_____ Gluc – glucose
_____ Bili – Bilirubin, total & direct	_____ Hgb – hemoglobin
_____ BMP – basic metabolic panel	_____ Lact – lactic acid/lactate
_____ BUN - Blood urea nitrogen	_____ Plt. Ct. – platelet count
_____ Lytes – electrolytes	_____ PT – prothrombin time
_____ CBC – complete blood count	_____ PTT – partial thromboplastin time
_____ Chol – cholesterol	_____ RPR – rapid plasma reagin
_____ ESR – erythrocyte sed rate	_____ T&S – type and screen
_____ EtOH - alcohol	_____ PSA – prostate specific antigen
_____ D-dimer	Other *blood cultures X 2*

SKILLS DRILL 11-2: WORD BUILDING (See Chapter 4, Medical Terminology)

Divide each of the words below into all of its elements (parts): prefix (P), word root (WR), combining vowel (CV), and suffix (S). Write the word part and its definition on the corresponding lines. Write the general meaning of the word in the space provided. If the word does not have a particular element, write NA (not applicable) in its place.

Example: thyrotoxicosis

Elements   _____ / ____*thyr*____ / ___*o*___ / ___*toxic*___ / ____*osis*_____
              P   WR   CV   WR   S

Definitions _____ / ____*thyroid*___ / _____ / ___*toxic*___ / __*abnormal condition*__

Meaning: abnormal condition of a toxic thyroid gland

1. bacteremia

   Elements   _____ / _____ / _____ / _____
                 P   WR   CV   S

   Definitions _____ / _____ / _____ / _____

   Meaning:

2. hypoglycemic

   Elements   _____ / _____ / _____ / _____ / _____
                 P   CV   WR   CV   S

   Definitions _____ / _____ / _____ / _____ / _____

   Meaning:

3. anaerobic

   Elements   _____ / _____ / _____ / _____ / _____
                 P   CV   WR   CV   S

   Definitions _____ / _____ / _____ / _____ / _____

   Meaning:

4. antibiotic

   Elements   _____ / _____ / _____ / _____ / _____
                 P   CV   WR   CV   S

   Definitions _____ / _____ / _____ / _____ / _____

   Meaning:

5. antimicrobial

   Elements   _____ / _____ / _____ / _____ / _____
                 P   CV   WR   CV   S

   Definitions _____ / _____ / _____ / _____ / _____

   Meaning:

6. gastrointestinal

   Elements   _____ / _____ / _____ / _____ / _____
                 WR   CV   WR   CV   S

   Definitions _____ / _____ / _____ / _____ / _____

   Meaning:

7. amniocentesis

   Elements   _____ / _____ / _____ / _____
                 P   WR   CV   S

   Definitions _____ / _____ / _____ / _____

   Meaning:

SKILLS DRILL 11-3: BLOOD CULTURE SPECIMEN COLLECTION

Instructions: Match the rationale with the corresponding step in the procedure.

Procedure Step

1. _____ Identify venipuncture site and release tourniquet.

2. _____ Aseptically select and assemble equipment.

3. _____ Perform friction scrub as prescribed.

4. _____ Allow site to air-dry.

5. _____ Cleanse the culture bottle stoppers while the site is drying.

6. _____ Mark the minimum and maximum fill on the culture bottles.

7. _____ Reapply tourniquet and perform venipuncture without touching the site.

8. _____ Inoculate the media bottles as required.

9. _____ Label the specimen containers with required ID, including the site of collection.

Rationale

A. Antisepsis does not occur instantly.

B. Notation of site location is necessary because there may be an isolated infection in that area.

C. Ensuring antiseptic technique and sterility of the site is critical to accurate diagnosis.

D. The CLSI standard states that the tourniquet should not be left on longer than 1 minute.

E. Inoculation of the medium can occur directly into the bottle or after collection when a syringe is used.

F. Blood culture bottles have vacuum, but it is not always measured as in evacuated tubes.

G. Aseptic technique reduces the risk of false positives due to contamination.

H. The tops of the culture bottles must be free of contaminants when they are inoculated.

I. Bacteria exist on the skin surface and can be removed temporarily.

SKILLS DRILL 11-4: BLOOD BANK ID, LABELING, AND SPECIMEN REQUIREMENTS

1. What types of collection tubes could be used? What type of tube is most often used?

_____

_____

_____

2. List four reasons why blood bank collection tubes might be rejected.

1. _____

2. _____

3. _____

4. _____

3. How long is a BB band on a patient's arm valid. How is that calculated?

_____

_____

_____

4. The Joint Commission's National Patient Safety Goal 01.01.01 states:

_____

_____

_____

5. Why does a "blood recipient patient ID system allow for one-person verification for blood transfusions?

_____

_____

_____

6. The nurse who is going to administer a blood transfusion initiates the validation for a patient by gathering four key facts about the blood product in the presence of the patient, and they are:

1. _____

2. _____

3. _____

4. _____

7. Why is a grossly hemolyzed sample not acceptable for BB testing?

_____

_____

_____

8. If you must collect a BB specimen and the patient has an IV, what additional responsibilities does the phlebotomist have at that time?

_____

_____

_____

SKILLS DRILL 11-5: TB TEST ADMINISTRATION (Text Procedure Box 11–4)

Instructions: Using the TEXTBOOK, fill in the blanks with the missing information.

Step	**Rationale**
1. Identify the patient, (A) _____ the procedure, and sanitize hands	Correct ID is vital to patient safety and meaningful test results. Proper hand hygiene plays a major role in infection control by protecting the phlebotomist, patient, and others from contamination. Gloves are sometimes put on at this point. Follow facility protocol.
2. Support the patient's arm on a firm surface and select a suitable site on the (B) _____ of the forearm, (C) _____ the antecubital crease.	The arm must be supported to minimize movement during test administration. Areas with scars, bruises, burns, rashes, excessive hair, or superficial veins must be avoided as they can interfere with (D) _____ of the test.
3. Clean the site with an (E) _____ pad and allow it to air dry.	Cleaning with antiseptic and allowing it to air dry permits maximum antiseptic action.
4. Put on gloves at this point if you have not already done so.	Gloves are necessary for safety and infection control.
5. Clean the top of the antigen bottle and draw (F) _____ of diluted antigen into the syringe.	The top of the bottle must be clean to prevent (G) _____ of the antigen.

6. Stretch the skin (H) _____ with the thumb in a manner similar to venipuncture and slip the needle just under the skin at a very (I) _____ _____ (approximately 10 to 15 degrees).

The skin must be taut, so that the needle will slip into it easily. The antigen must be injected just (J) _____ _____ _____ for accurate interpretation of results.

7. Pull (K) _____ on the syringe plunger slightly to make certain a vein has not been entered.

The antigen must not be injected into a vein.

8. Slowly expel the contents of the syringe to create a distinct, pale elevation commonly called a bleb or (L) _____.

9. Without applying pressure or gauze to the site, withdraw the needle, activate safety feature, and discard the needle.

Appearance of the bleb or wheal is a (M) _____ that the antigen has been injected properly.
Applying pressure could force the (N) _____ out of the site. Gauze might absorb the antigen. Both actions could invalidate test results. Activation of safety features and prompt needle disposal minimizes the chance of an accidental needlestick.
A bandage can absorb the fluid or cause irritation, resulting in misinterpretation of test results.

10. Ensure that the arm remains extended until the site has time to close. Do (O) _____ _____ a bandage.

11. Check the site for a reaction in (P) _____. This is called "reading" the reaction.

Maximum reaction is achieved in 48 to 72 hours. A reaction can be underestimated if read after this time.

12. Measure (Q) _____ (hardness) and interpret the result. Do not measure erythema (redness).
    Negative: induration absent or less than 5 mm in diameter.
    Doubtful: induration between 5 and 9 mm in diameter.
    Positive: induration (S) _____ _____ in diameter.

A TB reaction is interpreted according to the amount of induration or firm raised area due to (R) _____. A health status and age of the individual are important considerations when interpreting results.
5 mm of induration can be considered a positive test result in patients who are immunosuppressed due to chronic medical conditions.

SKILLS DRILL 11-6: PREGNANCY TEST PROCEDURE

Instructions: Match the rationale with the corresponding step in the procedure.

Procedure Step

1. _____ Identify the patient according to facility policy.

2. _____ Label the specimen cup with the patient's label.

3. _____ Obtain the patient's urine specimen.

4. _____ Remove the test device from the protective pouch and place it on a flat surface.

5. _____ Using the disposable dropper provided, add 3 drops of sample to the cassette well.

6. _____ Set a timer for the time the kit's manufacturer states a negative test must be read.

7. _____ Read the cassette window's results when the timer goes off.

Rationale

A. To avoid errors, label the specimen even if it is the only one being tested at that time.

B. For correct results, the urine must flow evenly onto the testing surface of the device.

C. The reaction time must be carefully timed and *not read* after 10 minutes.

D. The size of the drops must be exactly as specified and consistent for results to be accurate.

E. Correct ID is vital to patient safety and meaningful test results.

F. If the patient will be collecting a urine specimen at your testing site, explain how to do so.

G. A positive result can be read as soon as lines at both the T and C areas of the test cassette window appear.

Crossword

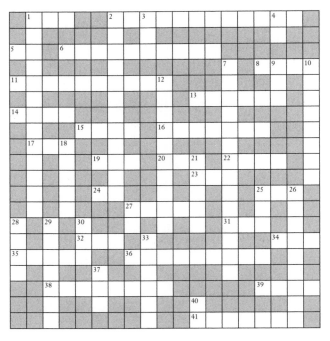

ACROSS

1. Coagulation test to monitor heparin therapy
2. Increased blood potassium
5. Scientific symbol for mercury
6. Blood types that are suitable to mix
8. BAC tests for this type of alcohol (abbrev)
11. Blood donated by people who will use it themselves
13. Another name for occult blood testing
14. Institute interested in curbing drug abuse and addition
15. Traceable component in Lookback program (abbrev)
16. Blood bank identification system
17. Type of antimicrobial resin
19. Initials used for a heart attack
20. Fluid around spinal column (abbrev.)
22. Type of Hgb that is measured in blood plasma
23. QC built into the instrument (abbrev.)
24. Checks to ensure that testing is done properly (abbrev.)
25. Agency that regulates blood products
27. Body fluid excreted by kidneys
31. Approx. number of gestational weeks for peak HCG levels
32. Cardiac protein specific for heart muscle
34. IL instrument that screens for renal disease
35. POC multi-test-panel chemistry analyzer
36. What i-STAT testing chip is called
38. Type of glucose meter
39. Org. sets guidelines for blood centers (abbrev)
41. BC media bottle used to grow microbes needing air

DOWN

1. Process of clumping together (i.e., Ag–Ab reaction)
2. Pertaining to a low glucose level
3. Partial thromboplastin time
4. Identification (abbrev.)
7. Strict protocol for forensic specimens
9. Tight glycemic index
10. Another name for small, portable POC instruments
12. Condition of microorganisms and toxins in the blood
18. Volunteer who gives blood for another person's use
21. Body discharge used to test for occult blood
25. Name of charcoal antimicrobial resin bottle (abbrev.)
26. BC media bottle used to grow microbes without air
27. Urinalysis (abbrev.)
28. Federal law that states qualifications for POCT personnel
29. A 9:1 ratio of blood to this anticoagulant is required
30. Extended test used to diagnose carbohydrate metabolism issues (abbrev.)
33. Generic name for grouping of commonly ordered tests
37. POCT kidney function test (abbrev)
40. One of the electrolytes measured by POC instruments

Chapter Review Questions

1. The fasting specimen for a GTT is drawn:
   a. as close to 6:00 A.M. as possible.
   b. before the test has actually begun.
   c. right after the glucose drink is finished.
   d. when the timing for the test begins.

2. Which of the following tube additives is preferred for the collection of a blood culture specimen?
   a. Citrate phosphate dextrose
   b. Sodium or potassium heparin
   c. Sodium polyanethol sulfonate
   d. Potassium oxalate and fluoride

3. TDM trough concentration may be defined as the:
   a. highest concentration of the drug during a dosing interval.
   b. lowest concentration of the drug during a dosing interval.
   c. maximum effectiveness of the drug in the tissues.
   d. none of the above.

4. In performing a glucose tolerance test, the fasting specimen is drawn at 6:15 A.M. and the patient finishes the glucose beverage at 6:30 A.M. When should the 2-hour specimen be collected?
   a. 8:15
   b. 8:30
   c. 9:15
   d. 9:30

5. Typical labeling requirements for a blood bank specimen include:
   a. full name of the physician who ordered the crossmatch
   b. hospital ID number only, no other identifier is accepted
   c. patient's date of birth and date and time of collection
   d. patient's first and last name, no middle initial needed

6. Withdrawing a unit of blood from a patient for therapeutic purposes is used as a treatment for:
   a. bacteremia.
   b. polycythemia
   c. major surgery.
   d. all of the above.

7. During a GTT, which of the following is acceptable?
   a. Allowing the patient to drink water at any time during the test
   b. Giving coffee to the patient after drawing the fasting specimen
   c. Permitting the patient to chew sugarless gum and smoke
   d. Timing all specimen collection after the fasting specimen was collected

8. A stool specimen is needed for the _____ test.
   a. A1 c
   b. Lipid
   c. Guaiac
   d. Strep

9. For what purpose is the Oral Glucose Challenge test used?
   a. To assess kidney and bladder function
   b. To check for lactose intolerance
   c. To detect absorption function disorders
   d. To screen for gestational diabetes

10. Autologous donation is performed to:
    a. avoid a transfusion reaction.
    b. save time in surgery.
    c. correct polycythemia.
    d. prevent stress on the heart.

11. Glycosylated hemoglobin is performed to monitor the effectiveness of therapy in which of the following conditions?
    a. Acidosis
    b. Diabetes
    c. Inflammation
    d. Renal disease

12. Prior to performing a test on a POCT instrument, the phlebotomist should:
    a. be able to operate the instrument correctly.
    b. be familiar with the instrument's maintenance procedures.
    c. understand the quality assurance aspects of the instrument.
    d. all of the above.

13. According to American Red Cross, persons wishing to donate blood must be:
    a. a resident of the state for at least 3 years.
    b. at least 17 years old in most of the states.
    c. fasting for 8 to 12 hours before arriving
    d. no less than 120 pounds and ambulatory

14. Which of the following procedures is required for a BC using a Chloroprep kit?
    a. Cleansing bottle tops with isopropyl alcohol
    b. Isopropyl swab before using Chloroprep
    c. Scrubbing for a full 2 minutes
    d. Using concentric circles with PVP

15. Blood bank specimens require which of the following identification information?
    a. Date and time of collection
    b. Patient's date of birth
    c. Patient's full name
    d. All of the above

16. The HemoCue Plasma/Low Hemoglobin instrument is used to indicate:

    a. iatrogenic anemia.

    b. hemolyzed red cells.

    c. kidney malfunction.

    d. respiratory distress.

17. Peak and trough specimens are collected for

    a. blood cultures times two.

    b. blood units to be cross-matched.

    c. cardiac enzyme evaluation.

    d. therapeutic drug monitoring.

18. In collecting blood cultures, one of the most frequent errors made is

    a. failure to inoculate two media bottles

    b. improper cleansing of the collection site

    c. incorrect labeling of the media bottles.

    d. not noting the venipuncture location.

19. Which of the following tests does not require special chain-of-custody documentation when collected?

    a. BAC

    b. Drug screen

    c. Paternity testing

    d. TDM

20. Which of the following POC tests is used to monitor warfarin therapy?

    a. ACT

    b. BN

    c. INR

    d. PTT

21. Pediatric blood cultures creates challenges because:

    a. BC collection requires two sets of cultures from one venipuncture

    b. most ill children have already received broad-spectrum antibiotics

    c. special media bottles are made to accommodate children's veins

    d. the antiseptic technique is different if you use Chloroprep swab

22. Hyperkalemia means:

    a. decreased calcium in the blood.

    b. increased calcium in the blood.

    c. increased potassium in the blood.

    d. increased sodium in the blood.

23. Postprandial refers to:

    a. after eating a meal.

    b. after fasting for 2 hours.

    c. just before eating.

    d. after medication.

24. In collecting a blood alcohol test for forensic purposes, the venipuncture site can be cleaned with:

    a. benzalkonium chloride.

    b. isopropyl alcohol.

    c. methyl alcohol.

    d. tincture of iodine.

25. Which of the following should be removed from a list of tests that the i-STAT instrument can measure?

    a. CBC and PT

    b. Hgb and Hct

    c. Gluc and BUN

    d. Na^+ and K^+

26. Blood levels of this specific analyte begin to rise within 4 hours of an MI.

    a. ALT

    b. TnT

    c. LDL

    d. BNP

27. When does the Lookback program occur?

    a. If there is a transfusion of incompatible blood to a patient

    b. At the time the unit is collected at the Blood Donor Center.

    c. When the blood service is made aware of a transfusion infection

    d. Before the blood unit is matched to a recipient's blood sample.

28. Molecular genetic testing requires:

    a. chain of custody protocol to be followed

    b. freezing of the spun sample immediately

    c. RNA tubes to be incubated at 37°C

    d. specimens to be collected in sterile EDTA

29. In the DOT's 10 Steps to Collection Site Security & Integrity, drug screen testing is secured for collection of the urine specimen because:

    a. employees must empty pockets and leave bags behind

    b. the collection site is inspected after completion

    c. the employee is closely observed by video camera

    d. the employee takes the specimen to the testing site

30. Monitoring the quality of waived testing being done at the bedside is a constant challenge for the laboratory because:

    a. more tests are classified as waived each year

    b. personnel doing waived testing are not trained

    c. quality control is not required for waived testing

    d. technology cannot keep up with big demand

Case Studies

Case Study 11-1: Prothrombin Test Collection

During clinical practicum, a phlebotomy student found that the requirements for drawing prothrombin times were not the same as he was taught in class. His clinical coordinator made it very clear that he was to follow facility protocol while he was in his clinical practicum. Therefore, when he was asked to collect a CBC and prothrombin time from a patient, he knew that the order of draw at this facility was citrate first, no discard tube. As he started to draw the specimen from the patient, he immediately ran into trouble when the vein rolled. He was certain that the needle had slipped beside the vein, so he tried to redirect it into the vein. After two unsuccessful redirects, the needle successfully entered the vein. He collected the citrate tube, followed by a lavender-top tube for the CBC. Later that day the coagulation department rejected the specimen and he was sent to re-collect it.

QUESTIONS

1. Why would the laboratory reject the sample?

2. What had the student done to cause the sample to be rejected?

3. How could the problem have been corrected while the needle was still in the arm?

Case Study 11-2: Blood Cultures and Butterflies

A phlebotomist was acting as preceptor for a phlebotomy student from the local college and was anxious to help her learn all the special tests that had not been practiced in class. When a stat blood culture and lytes on a patient in the ICU were ordered, the preceptor quickly grabbed the student and they headed for the floor. It was clear after looking at the patient that they would have to use a butterfly in a hand vein to collect the test specimens. The preceptor was busy helping the student prepare the site and, while setting out all of the equipment needed, he did not pay close attention to the order in which the media bottles were placed. The student was elated that she was able to access the difficult vein and that blood was flowing freely into the anaerobic bottle. After filling both it and the aerobic bottle to the proper level, she proceeded to draw an SST for electrolytes from the same site. The blood flow was now very slow, with blood entering the tube only a drop at a time. After patiently waiting for the tube to fill, both she and the preceptor were relieved to get finished. Almost immediately after returning to the laboratory and processing the sample, they were sent back to redraw the electrolytes because the potassium value was too high. Before leaving, the preceptor grabbed more BC equipment because he knew that the BCs would have to be redrawn also.

QUESTIONS

1. What had caused the potassium to be too high?

2. Why might they have expected this problem during the collection?

3. Why did the preceptor have the student redraw the BC also?

Case Study 11-3: Forensic Blood Alcohol Collection

In his first week on the job, a new graduate phlebotomist is called to the ER for a stat blood draw. When he arrives he is told to collect an ETOH. The patient smells heavily of alcohol and the phlebotomist is pretty certain that this is going to be an elevated ETOH with a legal investigation involved. The phlebotomist studied forensic blood alcohol collection in his training program, but this is the first real one he has collected and he is a little unsure of what to do. He remembers that a certain strict protocol is involved and that the site must not be cleaned with alcohol. All he has on his tray other than alcohol preps are a few benzalkonium chloride preps. He decides to use those. Laboratory protocol says to use an SST for an ETOH level, but he remembers something from his training about drawing a forensic ETOH in a gray top. He decides to draw one of each tube, collecting the SST first. A police officer arrives just as he is finishing and asks for the specimen in the gray-top tube and the accompanying paperwork. The phlebotomist feels relieved and returns to the laboratory.

QUESTIONS

1. Was the phlebotomist correct in deciding that the ETOH was going to involve an investigation, and what does a forensic collection involve?

2. What is the strict protocol that the phlebotomist remembered from his training and what does it involve?

3. Was benzalkonium chloride an acceptable antiseptic to use to collect the specimen?

4. Was it acceptable to draw both an SST and a gray top?

Chapter 12

Computers and Specimen Handling and Processing

Objectives

Study the information in the TEXTBOOK that corresponds to each objective to prepare yourself for the activities in this chapter.

1 Demonstrate basic knowledge of the elements of a computer system, define associated terminology and understand the flow of specimens through the laboratory information system.

2 Explain routine and special specimen handling procedures for laboratory specimens, and identify preanalytical errors that may occur during collection, labeling, transporting, and processing.

3 Describe the steps involved in processing the different types of specimens, time constraints, and exceptions for delivery and list the criteria for specimen rejection.

4 Define how bar codes are used in health care and list information found on a bar code computer label. Identify OSHA-required protective equipment worn when processing specimens.

Matching

Use choices only once unless otherwise indicated.

MATCHING 12-1: KEY TERMS AND DESCRIPTIONS

Match each key term with the *best* description.

Key Terms (1–20)

1. _____ Accession number
2. _____ Aerosol
3. _____ Aliquot
4. _____ Bar code
5. _____ Biobank
6. _____ Breach
7. _____ Central processing
8. _____ Centrifuge
9. _____ Cloud
10. _____ Cursor
11. _____ Data
12. _____ DOT
13. _____ EMR
14. _____ Hardware
15. _____ HIS
16. _____ IATA
17. _____ Icon
18. _____ ID code
19. _____ Input
20. _____ Interface

Descriptions

A. Area where specimens are received and prioritized for testing
B. Computer equipment used to process data
C. Connect for the purpose of interaction
D. Data Leak
E. Department of Transportation
F. Electronic medical records
G. Enter data into a computer
H. Fine mist of specimen
I. Flashing indicator on the computer screen
J. Hospital Information System
K. Image used to represent a program or function on a computer
L. Information collected for analysis or computation
M. International Air Transport Association
N. LIS number generated for a specimen when entered into the computer
O. Machine that spins blood and other specimens
P. Off-site hardware for unlimited data storage
Q. Parallel array of alternately spaced black bars and white spaces
R. Portion of a specimen used for testing
S. Repository where human biological samples are stored for research
T. Unique identification for a computer user

Key Terms (21–40)

21. _____ LIS
22. _____ Measurand
23. _____ Menu
24. _____ Middleware
25. _____ Mnemonic
26. _____ Network
27. _____ Output
28. _____ Password
29. _____ Preanalytical
30. _____ Precentrifugation
31. _____ Postcentrifugation

Descriptions

A. Application software often called "plumbing"
B. Computer screen and keyboard
C. Computers that are linked together for the purpose of sharing resources
D. Identification and tracking system using radio waves
E. Laboratory information system
F. List of options from which a user may choose
G. Memory-aiding codes
H. Place to preserve information outside of the CPU
I. Prior to testing a sample
J. Programming required to control computer hardware
K. Quantity not sufficient
L. Quantity of specimen intended to be measured
M. Random-access memory
N. Read-only memory

32. _____ QNS

33. _____ RAM

34. _____ RFID

35. _____ RNA

36. _____ ROM

37. _____ Software

38. _____ Storage

39. _____ Terminal

40. _____ USB drive

O. Return of processed information to user or someone in another location
P. Ribonucleic acid
Q. Secret code that uniquely identifies a person as system user
R. Time period after specimen centrifugation
S. Time period after specimen collection and before centrifugation
T. Universal Serial Bus device used for storing information

MATCHING 12-2: COMPUTER SKILL AND ACTIVITY PERFORMED

Match the computer skill with the activity performed.

Computer Skill

1. _____ Logging on

2. _____ Cursor movement

3. _____ Using icons

4. _____ Entering data

5. _____ Correcting errors

6. _____ Verifying data

7. _____ Making order inquiries

8. _____ Canceling orders

Activity Performed

The phlebotomist:
A. Looks up a test order and deletes or cancels it
B. Notes where indicator is flashing and enters information at that point
C. Presses the delete key and retypes the information
D. Proceeds to the computer and enters a password
E. Retrieves other test information ordered on the same patient
F. Reviews information, and chooses to modify, delete, or accept
G. Types in patient information and presses the Enter key, so it can be processed
H. Uses the mouse to click on a small image on the screen

MATCHING 12-3: COMPUTER EQUIPMENT AND COMPUTER ELEMENT

Match the computer equipment with the associated computer element. Choices may be used more than once.

Computer Equipment

1. _____ Bar code readers

2. _____ CDs

3. _____ Database systems

4. _____ External hard drives

5. _____ Graphics programs

6. _____ Handhelds

7. _____ Keyboards

8. _____ LIS

9. _____ Middleware

10. _____ Modems

11. _____ Monitors

12. _____ Printers

13. _____ Routers

14. _____ Scanners

15. _____ Spreadsheet programs

Computer Element

A. Hardware
B. Software
C. Storage

MATCHING 12-4: SPECIMEN AND TYPE OF PROCESSING

Match the specimen with the type of processing normally required. Choices may be used more than once.

Specimen

1. _____ Aldosterone in a red top

2. _____ Ammonia in a green top

3. _____ Blood culture in an SPS tube

4. _____ BMP in an SST

5. _____ CBC in a lavender top

6. _____ Copper in a nonadditive royal blue top

7. _____ CSF in a clear plastic tube

8. _____ Cyclosporine in a green top

9. _____ Electrolytes in a PST

10. _____ Glucose in an anticoagulant gray top

11. _____ Hemoglobin A1c in a purple top

12. _____ Hepatitis C qualitative RNA in a PPT

13. _____ PT in a light blue top

14. _____ Zinc in an EDTA royal blue top

15. _____ Urinalysis specimen

Type of Processing

A. Centrifuge after clotting
B. Centrifuge immediately
C. Do not centrifuge

Labeling Exercises

LABELING EXERCISE 12-1: COMPUTER WORK FLOW CHART (Text Fig. 12-5)

This flow chart describes the test requisition and specimen collection process. Fill in the missing flow chart words numbered 1 through 5 on the corresponding numbered lines. Then write the computer program name of each numbered box in the flow chart on the corresponding numbered line.

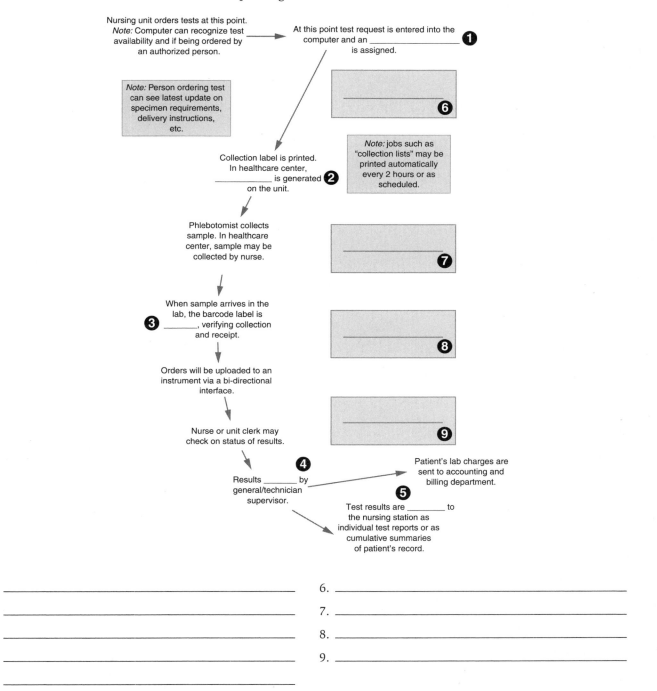

1. _____   6. _____

2. _____   7. _____

3. _____   8. _____

4. _____   9. _____

5. _____

LABELING EXERCISE 12-2: SPECIAL HANDLING

Use a blue pen or pencil to place a "C" next to the following specimens that must be chilled in ice slurry or cooling rack. Use a red pen or pencil to place a "W" next to specimens that must be kept warm at 37°C. Use a black pen or pencil to place a "P" next to specimens that must be protected from light.

Tests

1. _____ ACTH

2. _____ Ammonia

3. _____ Bilirubin

4. _____ Beta carotene

5. _____ Catecholamines

6. _____ Cold agglutinin

7. _____ Cryoglobulin

8. _____ Cryofibrinogen

9. _____ Gastrin

10. _____ Homocysteine

11. _____ Lactic acid

12. _____ PTH

13. _____ RNA-based tests

14. _____ Urine porphyrins

15. _____ Vitamin A

LABELING EXERCISE 12-3: PREANALYTICAL ERRORS

Examples of preanalytical errors are listed below. Write "PC" next to the preanalytical errors that happen prior to collection, "TC" next to errors that happen at the time of collection, "ST" next to errors that happen during specimen transport, "SP" next to errors that happen during specimen processing, and "SS" next to errors that happen during specimen storage. Some examples may have more than one correct answer.

Preanalytical Error Examples

1. _____ Dehydrated patient

2. _____ Duplicate test orders

3. _____ Evaporation

4. _____ Exposure to light

5. _____ Inadequate fast

6. _____ Incomplete centrifugation

7. _____ Incorrect collection tube

8. _____ Medications

9. _____ Mislabeled aliquot

10. _____ Nonsterile site preparation

11. _____ Patient stress

12. _____ Strenuous exercise

13. _____ Temperature change outside of defined limit

14. _____ Underfilled tube

15. _____ Vigorous mixing

16. _____ Wrong collection time

17. _____ Wrong order of draw

18. _____ Wrong test ordered

Knowledge Drills

KNOWLEDGE DRILL 12-1: CAUTION AND KEY POINT RECOGNITION

The following sentences are taken from "CAUTION and KEY POINT" statements found throughout Chapter 12 in the TEXTBOOK. Using the TEXTBOOK, fill in the blanks with the missing information.

1. (A) _____ (B) _____ makes sharing information so easy that (C) _____

   (D) _____ can be violated.

2. If a (A) _____ test is ordered with other analytes that require (B) _____, it should be

   collected in a (C) _____ (D) _____.

3. According to a 2013 article in the *Journal of Environmental and Public Health*, results of community outreach

   studies found that (A) _____ by erythrocytes and (B) _____ in blood specimens can

   falsely lower (C) _____ values from (D) _____ per hour.

4. It has been estimated that (A) _____ of all laboratory (B) _____ occur prior to

   (C) _____.

5. It is important to know the following temperatures related to specimen handling:

   Body temperature: (A) _____ (_____)

   Room temperature: (B) _____

   Refrigerated temperature: (C) _____

   Frozen temperature: (D) _____ or lower (some specimens require −70°C or lower)

6. (A) _____ regulations require those who process specimens to wear (B) _____

   (C) _____ (D) _____ (E) (_____), which includes gloves, fully closed,

   (F) _____-resistant lab coats or aprons, and protective face gear, such as mask and goggles with

   side (G) _____, or chin-length face shields.

7. Stoppers must be left on tubes while awaiting and during (A) _____ to prevent

   (B) _____, evaporation, (C) _____ (fine spray) formation, and (D) _____

   changes.

8. Because a centrifuge generates (A) _____ during operation, specimens requiring

   (B) _____ should be processed in a temperature-controlled (C) _____ centrifuge.

9. Sometimes the expression (A) _____ (B) _____ is used to describe how a specimen

   should be transported. What it really means is the specimen requires (C) _____ and should be

   transported in an (D) _____ (E) _____ or cooling rack.

10. Never put (A) _____ and (B) _____, or (C) _____ from specimens with

    different (D) _____ in the same aliquot tube.

11. There are different (A) _____ formulations, and some of them cannot be used for certain tests.

    For example: (B) _____, (C) _____ cannot be used for (D) _____ levels;

    ammonium (E) _____ cannot be used for ammonia levels; and sodium (F) _____

    cannot be used for sodium levels.

12. (A) _____ the serum or plasma into (B) _____ (C) _____ is not recom-

    mended because it increases the possibility of (D) _____ formation or (E) _____.

13. Tests that are seriously affected by (A) _____ include (B) _____, plasma free hemoglobin, (C) _____ and T, (D) _____, and (E) _____.

14. According to CLSI nonanticoagulant (A) _____ tubes should be placed in an (B) _____ (C) _____ as soon as they have been (D) _____.

15. Serum and plasma (A) _____ should not be (B) _____ and (C) _____ more than (D) _____.

KNOWLEDGE DRILL 12-2: SCRAMBLED WORDS

Unscramble the following words using the hints given in parenthesis and the letters that have been placed in the correct boxes. Finish writing the correct spelling of the scrambled word in the corresponding boxes.

1. cremtoup (health care tool)

		m		u			

2. dolttec (SSTs before they can be centrifuged)

	l			t		

3. fewtoras (coded instructions to control hardware)

			t	w			

4. legtangutia (some blood specimens do this at room temperature)

a				u					t	

5. paveroontia (concentrates analytes)

			p	o			i		

6. pratmeertue (can affect specimen integrity)

t				e		a				

7. scisyllogy (metabolic process)

		y		o		s		

8. sloymeshi (reason for specimen rejection)

	e				y			

9. teeptip (used to create an aliquot)

p		p				

10. inmalter (a monitor and a keyboard)

	e			i			

KNOWLEDGE DRILL 12-3: TRUE/FALSE

The following statements are all false. Circle the one or two words that make the statement false and write the correct word(s) that would make the statement true in the space provided.

1. To be considered computer literate, an individual must be able to perform complex operations using computers.

2. Congress took steps to eliminate confidentiality violations by enacting OSHA, which is designed to protect the privacy and security of patient information.

3. A computer screen and a CPU combination is called a "terminal"; these are necessary peripherals for most computers, and are found throughout the laboratory at workstations or directly connected to an analyzer.

4. While most point-of-care analyzers are interface capable, the decision to do so is based on the number of tests performed and the cost of the test to the patient.

5. Chilling a specimen maintains metabolic processes and stabilizes and protects analytes.

6. The most frequently cited reason for rejection of chemistry specimens is mislabeling, followed by insufficient amount of specimen, or QNS.

7. CLSI and OSHA guidelines require specimen transport bags to have a biohazard logo, a liquid-tight closure and a slip pocket for small tubes.

8. After collection, rough handling and agitation can hemolyze specimens, activate white cells, and affect coagulation tests as well as break the collection tubes.

9. Glucose test specimens drawn in sodium fluoride are stable for 48 hours at room temperature and up to 72 hours when refrigerated at 4°C to 8°C.

10. The most frequently cited reason for rejection of hematology specimens is hemolysis.

KNOWLEDGE DRILL 12-4: SPECIMEN REJECTION CRITERIA

The following are examples of specimen rejection criteria (Text Table 12–3). Fill in the blanks with the missing information.

1. Inadequate, (A) _____, or missing patient (B) _____ (e.g., (C) _____ specimen that is not (D) _____).

2. (A) _____ additive tube (e.g., (B) _____ specimen in a (C) _____ filled light blue top tube lacks required (D) _____ to additive (D) _____).

3. Hemolysis (e.g., (A) _____ (B) _____ specimen).

4. Wrong (A) _____ (e.g., CBC collected in a (B) _____ top tube).

5. (A) _____ tube (e.g., specimen collected in a tube that (B) _____ a month ago).

6. (A) _____ in the specimen (e.g., CBC that was not (B) _____ (C) _____).

7. (A) _____ specimen (e.g., urine C & S in an (B) _____ container).

8. (A) _____ (quantity not sufficient) (e.g., partially filled (B) _____ submitted for (C) _____ chemistry tests that require a (D) _____ of 1 mL serum).

9. Wrong collection (A) _____ (e.g., (B) _____ (C) _____ monitoring (D) (_____) specimen collected before the drug was given).

10. Exposure to (A) _____ (e.g., (B) _____ specimen that was not protected from (C) _____).

11. Delay in (A) _____ (e.g., (B) _____ specimen in an EDTA tube received 5 hours after it was (C) _____).

12. Delay in (A) _____ (e.g., (B) _____ specimen that was not (C) _____ from the (D) _____ until 4 hours after collection).

13. Body temperature (A) (_____) requirement not met (e.g., (B) _____ (C) _____ specimen delivered at room temperature).

14. Chilling requirement not met (e.g. (A) _____ specimen delivered at (B) _____ temperature).

15. Specimen (A) _____ affected by (B) _____ (e.g., potassium or (C) _____ specimen arrives on (D) _____).

Skills Drills

SKILLS DRILL 12-1: REQUISITION ACTIVITY

Any Hospital USA
1123 West Physician Drive
Any Town USA

Laboratory Test Requisition

– –

PATIENT INFORMATION:

Name: _____ Doe _____ Jane _____ A _____
                 (last)   (first)   (MI)

Identification Number: __713562941__   Birth Date: __04/23/40__

Referring Physician: __Bright, Samuel__

Date to be Collected: __08/11/2015__   Time to be Collected: __0600__

Special Instructions: _____

– –

TEST(S) ORDERED:

Chemistry		Coagulation	
	NH4 – Ammonia		D-dimer
√	Bili – Bilirubin, total & direct	√	PT – prothrombin time
	BMP – basic metabolic panel		PTT – partial thromboplastin time
	BUN - Blood urea nitrogen	**Hematology**	
	Chol – cholesterol		CBC – (complete blood count)
	EtOH - alcohol		ESR – (erythrocyte sed rate)
	Gluc – glucose		Hgb – (hemoglobin)
	Lytes – electrolytes		H & H (hemoglobin & Hematocrit)
	Lact – lactic acid/lactate		RBC (Red blood cell count)
	PSA – prostatic specific antigen		WBC (White blood cell count)
Other	√ Cold agglutinin		

A phlebotomist collected specimens for this requisition and delivered them to the specimen processing. One specimen was wrapped in foil; one was in a 37°C heat block, and one was a normal draw light-blue–top tube with no special handling that was about two-thirds full with a note attached stating that it was a difficult draw. The specimens were correctly labeled. Assuming the specimens were handled properly:

1. Which specimen was wrapped in foil? Why? What process does the foil prevent? _____

_____

2. Which specimen was in the heat block? Why? _____

_____

3. Which specimen was in the light blue top? Why? _____

_____

4. Should the light blue top be accepted for testing? Why or why not? _____

_____

SKILLS DRILL 12-2: WORD BUILDING

Divide each of the words below into all of its elements (parts); prefix (P), word root (WR), combining vowel (CV), and suffix (S). Write the word part and its definition on the corresponding lines. Write the general meaning of the word in the space provided. If the word does not have a particular element, write NA (not applicable) in its place.

Example: phlebotomy

Elements _____ /_____*phleb*_____ /___*o*___ /_____*tomy*_____
                              P   WR   CV   S

Definitions _____ /_____*vein*_____ /_____ /__*cutting/incision*__

Meaning: cutting or incision of a vein

1. glycolysis

    Elements _____ /_____ /_____ /_____
                                  P   WR   CV   S

    Definitions _____ /_____ /_____ /_____

    Meaning:

2. cryofibrinogen

    Elements _____ /_____ /_____ /_____ /_____
                                  WR   CV   WR   CV   S

    Definitions _____ /_____ /_____ /_____ /_____

    Meaning:

3. diagnosis

    Elements _____ /_____ /_____ /_____
                                  P   WR   CV   S

    Definitions _____ /_____ /_____ /_____

    Meaning:

4. terminology

    Elements _____ /_____ /_____ /_____
                                  P   WR   CV   S

    Definitions _____ /_____ /_____ /_____

    Meaning:

5. mnemonic

    Elements _____ /_____ /_____ /_____
                                  P   WR   CV   S

    Definitions _____ /_____ /_____ /_____

    Meaning:

6. preanalytical

    Elements _____ /_____ /_____ /_____
                                  P   WR   CV   S

    Definitions _____ /_____ /_____ /_____

    Meaning:

Crossword

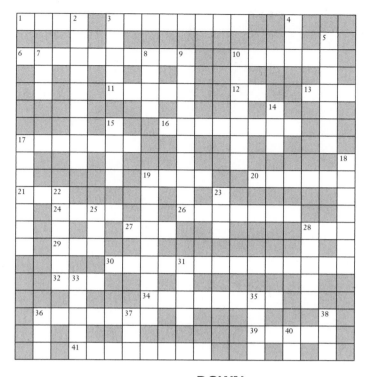

ACROSS

1. Information that has been collected for analysis
3. Another name for the sample being tested
6. Of or relating to electrons
10. Fluid portion of living blood
11. Electronic equipment used to connect computers by telephone line
12. Identification (abbrev.)
13. Time from collection to result (abbrev.)
16. Process of using a mechanical device made to duplicate human function
17. Blood spray when tube stopper is removed
19. List of options from which the user may choose
20. To form into ice
21. Less than the amount needed (abbrev.)
24. Computer terminal is called _____ ware
26. Place for keeping data, e.g., USB drive
27. Electronic medical record
28. Cardiopulmonary resuscitation
29. Estimated time of arrival
30. Process of spinning blood tube at high rpms
32. Test for diffuse coagulation throughout the body (abbrev.)
34. Device that computes
36. Method of doing something in stepwise procedure
39. Collection vials
41. Coded instructions to control hardware

DOWN

2. Enter specimen request into computer
3. Fluid in a clotted tube
4. Computer software system used in the laboratory (abbrev.)
5. Crucial consideration when loading a centrifuge
7. Local interconnected computer network
8. An individual computer station
9. The three basic _____ of a computer system
10. Computer peripheral used to create hard copies
14. Substance used to make slurry for chilling specimens
15. Bar _____
17. Portion of specimen used for testing
18. Anticoagulant in green top tube
19. Memory-aiding abbreviations
22. Protective covering or structure
23. Read-only memory (abbrev.)
25. Ribonucleic acid (abbrev.)
28. Make specimen cold to slow down metabolic processes
31. Way to measure centrifuge speed (abbrev.)
33. Images used to request appropriate computer functions
35. Anticoagulant in lavender tubes
36. Plasma tubes with separator gel (abbrev.)
37. Serum tubes with separator gel (abbrev.)
38. Test measuring rate of RBC sedimentation (abbrev.)
40. Company that manufactures collection equipment (abbrev.)

Chapter Review Questions

1. The abbreviation for computer memory that can be lost if not saved is:
   a. RAM.   c. RIM.
   b. REM.   d. ROM.

2. Normal operation of a computer is controlled by:
   a. applications software.
   b. hardware.
   c. storage memory.
   d. systems software.

3. Input devices include:
   a. cursors.   c. icons.
   b. glidepads.   d. monitors.

4. This device automatically resets itself at the correct point for data input after the Enter key is pressed.
   a. CPU   c. icon
   b. cursor   d. ROM

5. A specimen is delivered to a laboratory that has an LIS, the very next step is to:
   a. assign it an accession number.
   b. order and print a collection label.
   c. scan the bar code for verification.
   d. send the charge for it to billing

6. Information in the form of alternately spaced black bars and white spaces is called a/an:
   a. accession number.   c. ID code.
   b. bar code.   d. mnemonic.

7. The abbreviation of the organization that was established to ensure that POC analyzers are able to talk to any LIS is:
   a. CIC.   c. DOT.
   b. CLIA.   d. IATA.

8. Results of a bilirubin test specimen exposed to light for an hour can be decreased up to:
   a. 10%.   c. 50%.
   b. 25%.   d. 65%.

9. Glycolysis can falsely lower glucose values at a rate of up to:
   a. 1% to 3% per hour   c. 5% to 7% per hour
   b. 3% to 5% per hour   d. 6% to 10% per hour

10. Inadequate mixing of an anticoagulant tube can lead to:
    a. cell decomposition
    b. extreme hemolysis.
    c. immediate glycolysis.
    d. microclot formation.

11. Average normal body temperature is:
    a. 20°F.   c. 37°F.
    b. 37°C.   d. 98.6°C.

12. The specimen for this test should not be chilled.
    a. Ammonia   c. Lactic acid
    b. Homocysteine   d. Potassium

13. To "balance" a centrifuge means to:
    a. fill it completely with tubes that are all of the same specimen type.
    b. place it on a sturdy countertop with a level and motionless surface.
    c. put tubes of equal size and amount of specimen opposite each other.
    d. all of the above.

14. Which of the following actions by a specimen processor violates OSHA regulations?
    a. Loading specimens into the centrifuge without wearing gloves
    b. Pouring specimens into aliquot tubes instead of using pipettes
    c. Wearing an unfastened lab coat while creating specimen aliquots
    d. All of the above

15. Latent fibrin formation in serum can result from:
    a. a centrifuge speed that is set too high.
    b. a long delay before centrifugation.
    c. gross hemolysis of the specimen.
    d. incomplete clotting when centrifuged.

16. Which specimen should not be centrifuged?
    a. CBC   c. Protime
    b. Glucose   d. Vitamin B_{12}

17. Which of the following would most likely be rejected for testing?
    a. Bilirubin specimen in a half-filled microtube
    b. CBC specimen in a slightly underfilled tube
    c. Hemolyzed specimen for potassium testing
    d. UA specimen in a container that is not sterile

18. Which specimen may take longer than normal to clot?
    a. Chilled specimen that is from an outpatient clinic
    b. Specimen from a patient on anticoagulant therapy
    c. Specimen from a patient with a high WBC count
    d. All of the above

19. According to CLSI this test is negatively affected by tube system transportation.
    a. albumin
    b. creatinine
    c. potassium
    d. uric acid

20. A blood specimen aliquot can remain at room temperature no longer than:
    a. 1 hour
    b. 2 hours
    c. 4 hours
    d. 8 hours

21. The difference between bar codes and radio frequency identification is:
    a. Radio frequency ID is less expensive.
    b. Radio frequency ID is not standardized.
    c. RFID can work up to 100 feet away.
    d. RFID cannot be used to label specimens.

22. Most POC analyzers are interface capable, but the decision to do so is based on the:
    a. cost of the test that is being performed.
    b. impact the test result has on the patient.
    c. number of analyzers that are available.
    d. type of POCT instrument being used.

23. Specimens transported by a courier must:
    a. be kept close to body temperature.
    b. centrifuged prior to transportation.
    c. protected from direct sun exposure.
    d. transported horizontally for safety.

24. Which two federal agencies work together to regulate the transporting of biological specimens off site?
    a. CAP and CLSI
    b. CLIA and IATA
    c. DOT and IATA
    d. FDA and OSHA

25. When thawing a frozen sample, the procedure is to:
    a. heat it in a warm water bath; invert it occasionally.
    b. thaw it in the refrigerator; mix only when thawed.
    c. warm it at 25°C; invert 10 to 20 times after thawing.
    d. warm it at 37°C; mixing it when ready for testing.

Case Studies

Case Study 12-1: Specimen Handling and Collection Verification

Chad is the lone phlebotomist on the night shift at a hospital. At 03:00 he collects a timed glucose using a PST per laboratory policy. On return to the laboratory he attempts to verify collection of the specimen. The LIS is down for scheduled updates but will be back on-line soon. He sets the tube in a rack of extra tubes collected during ER draws. He intends to verify collection in a few minutes but starts sorting morning draw requisitions and forgets about it. After that he goes on break and loses track of time reading a newspaper until he is paged by an ER nurse to collect a STAT CBC. He tries but is unable to collect it, so an ER tech collects it while starting an IV. It is past time for Chad's shift to be over, so he quickly grabs the tube, labeling it on the way back to the laboratory. The 07:00 shift is already there. One of them has just returned from trying to collect a glucose specimen because the patient's nurse had called for results and there was no record of the draw. The patient insisted he had already been drawn, and refused to be drawn again. Chad remembers the glucose specimen in the rack. He quickly verifies collection of it and the STAT and personally delivers them to the proper laboratory departments. The chemistry tech refuses to accept the glucose specimen. When the STAT CBC is tested, microclots are detected, and it has to be recollected.

QUESTIONS

1. Why do you think the glucose specimen was rejected for testing?

2. What could Chad have done differently, so the specimen would not have been forgotten?

3. What do you think caused the microclots in the CBC?

4. How should Chad have handled the CBC?

Case Study 12-2: Specimen Rejection and Centrifuge Operation

Melinda, a recent phlebotomy graduate, works with an experienced phlebotomist in a clinic. Her job involves drawing specimens, centrifuging them if required, and sending them by courier to an off-site laboratory. Today her coworker is ill, and Melinda is by herself. Quite a few patients arrived shortly after the clinic opened at 08:00, but most were easy draws and by 09:15 only three are left. The first one, an elderly man, needs a PT and BMP. She draws a light blue top and SST. The next one needs a liver profile. He is a difficult draw and her first attempt is unsuccessful. On the second try blood flows slowly, but she is able to collect a few milliliters in an SST before it stops. The last patient needs a homocysteine level. She easily draws the specimen. The waiting room is empty. She looks at the clock. It is 09:40. The courier arrives in 20 minutes and she has not centrifuged any of the specimens. She quickly loads the centrifuge and turns it on. It makes a terrible noise, so she turns it off. She moves a few tubes around and starts it again. This time it sounds OK and finishes spinning just as the courier arrives. She quickly grabs the tubes. As she puts them in a transport bag, she notices the serum in one SST looks gelled. She wonders why but puts it in the bag anyway. The courier takes the bag and leaves. The elderly man's BMP specimen, the difficult draw specimen, and the homocysteine specimen are all rejected by the laboratory and must be recollected.

QUESTIONS

1. Why do you think the centrifuge made the noise? Why did moving tubes fix the problem?

2. What do you think the gel-like substance in the elderly man's BMP specimen was? What may have caused it, and would that be why it was rejected for testing?

3. What do you think was most likely wrong with the difficult draw specimen?

4. Why do you think the homocysteine specimen was rejected?

Case Study 12-3: Specimen Processing Issues

Janine, a phlebotomist has been newly trained to do specimen processing in the hospital laboratory. She is normally expected to work alongside an experienced processor except when that person is on break or at lunch. Today, while the other processor was on his lunch break, multiple specimens arrived from a new off-site drawing station. All of the specimens had proper identification and paperwork. One of them, an ACTH specimen was in a cooling rack. There were several serum separator tubes (SSTs) that had already been centrifuged. The gel had formed at a slant in all of them. She examined each of them very closely. In addition, there were several other SSTs that had not been centrifuged. The clot was stuck to the tube stopper in every one of these tubes. Janine eventually accessioned all of the specimens, loaded the unspun SSTs and the ACTH into the centrifuge, started it up, and began preparing to aliquot the SSTs that had already been spun. Just then the centrifuge began vibrating loudly and turned itself off.

QUESTIONS

1. Should Janine have rejected any of the specimens? Why or why not?

2. What could have caused the gel to form at a slant in the SSTs, and why do you think Janine examined them so closely?

3. What can cause clotted blood to stick to tube stoppers? How can this be prevented?

4. One specimen was handled incorrectly. Which one was it and how should it have been handled?

5. What do you think caused the centrifuge to vibrate loudly and shut itself off. What should Janine do about that?

Chapter 13
Nonblood Specimens and Tests

Objectives

Study the information in your TEXTBOOK that corresponds to each objective to prepare yourself for the activities in this chapter.

1 Demonstrate knowledge of nonblood specimens and tests, and define associated terminology.

2 Describe collection, labeling, and handling procedures for nonblood specimens.

Matching

Use choices only once unless otherwise indicated.

MATCHING 13-1: KEY TERMS AND DESCRIPTIONS

Match each key term with the *best* description.

Key Terms (1–15)

1. _____ AFP
2. _____ Amniotic fluid
3. _____ Buccal swab
4. _____ C&S
5. _____ C difficile
6. _____ Catheterized
7. _____ Clean-catch
8. _____ CSF
9. _____ Expectorate
10. _____ FIT
11. _____ FOBT
12. _____ Gastric analysis
13. _____ *H. pylori*
14. _____ Iontophoresis
15. _____ Midstream

Descriptions

A. Antigen in amniotic fluid measured to assess fetal development
B. Bacteria that can cause chronic gastritis and lead to peptic ulcer disease
C. Contains material collected from the inside of the cheek
D. Cough up and spit out mucus or phlegm
E. Detects hidden blood in feces
F. Fluid from the space surrounding the spinal cord
G. Frequent causative agent of hospital-acquired diarrhea
H. Growing and determining the antibiotic susceptibility of a microbe
I. Liquid from the sac that surrounds and cushions a fetus
J. Method of obtaining an uncontaminated urine sample
K. Method used to stimulate sweat production
L. Occult blood test that detects globin from human hemoglobin
M. Test that evaluates stomach acid production
N. Urine specimen collected from tubing inserted into the bladder
O. Urine specimen obtained during the middle of urination

Key Terms (16–30)

16. _____ NP
17. _____ O&P
18. _____ Occult blood
19. _____ PCR
20. _____ Pericardial fluid
21. _____ Peritoneal fluid
22. _____ Pleural fluid
23. _____ Serous fluid
24. _____ Sputum
25. _____ Suprapubic
26. _____ Sweat chloride
27. _____ Synovial fluid
28. _____ 24-hour urine
29. _____ UA
30. _____ UTI

Descriptions

A. Blood hidden from the naked eye
B. Fecal test for parasites and their eggs
C. Fluid from the abdominal cavity
D. Fluid from the lung cavity
E. Fluid from the sac surrounding the heart
F. Infection in the urinary tract
G. Joint fluid
H. Mucus coughed up from the trachea or lungs
I. Pale yellow serum-like fluid
J. Refers to the nasal cavity and pharynx
K. Routine urine test
L. Test used in the diagnosis of cystic fibrosis
M. Testing process that can detect and amplify DNA
N. Type of pooled urine specimen
O. Urine specimen aspirated through the bladder wall

MATCHING 13-2: NONBLOOD TEST AND TYPE OF SPECIMEN

Match the test to the type of specimen that may be required.

Nonblood Test

1. _____ AFP

2. _____ Biopsy

3. _____ C-UBT

4. _____ Diphtheria culture

5. _____ DNA analysis

6. _____ Guaiac

7. _____ HCG

8. _____ Male fertility studies

9. _____ Strep culture

10. _____ TB culture

Type of Specimen

A. Amniotic fluid
B. Breath
C. Buccal swab
D. Feces
E. NP swab
F. Semen
G. Sputum
H. Throat swab
I. Tissue
J. Urine

MATCHING 13-3: NONBLOOD TEST AND TEST EQUIPMENT, PROCEDURE, OR SPECIMEN REQUIREMENTS

Match each of the following nonblood tests to the equipment, procedure, or specimen requirement listed.

Nonblood Test

1. _____ CSF analysis

2. _____ C-urea breath test

3. _____ DNA analysis

4. _____ Gastric analysis

5. _____ NP culture

6. _____ Occult blood

7. _____ Pregnancy test

8. _____ Sweat chloride

9. _____ Urine C&S

10. _____ Urine chemical analysis

Test Equipment, Procedure, or Specimen Requirements

A. Buccal swab
B. Concentrated urine specimen
C. Cotton or Dacron-tipped flexible wire swab
D. Histamine or pentagastrin as a stimulant
E. Machine with electrodes to stimulate the skin
F. Special Mylar balloons
G. Reagent strip
H. Designated test card
I. Sterile collection container
J. Three or four sterile tubes

Labeling Exercises

LABELING EXERCISE 13-1: SPECIMEN COLLECTION DEVICES AND CONTAINERS

Label the photo of each specimen collection device or container shown below with the name of a test specimen that is collected in it. Choose from the following list of tests.

Tests

AFB culture
Creatinine clearance
CSF analysis
DNA
Fecal fat O&P
Strep culture
UA (infant)
UA (off-site analysis)
Urine C&S

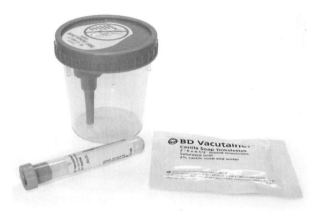

1. _____

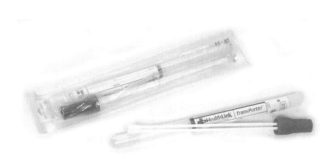

2. _____

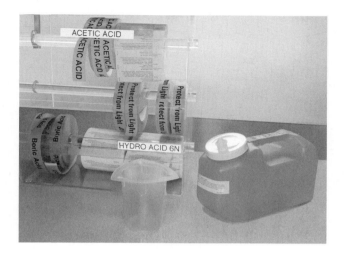

3. _____

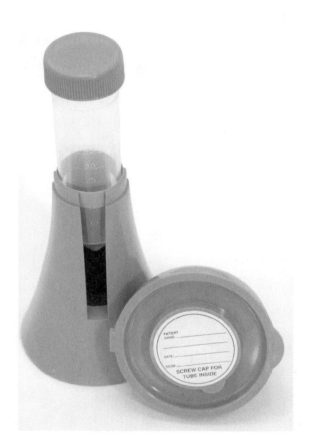

4. _____

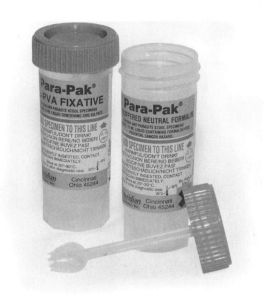

5. _____

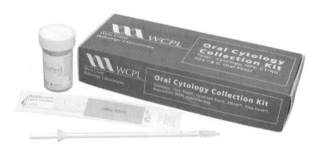

6. _____

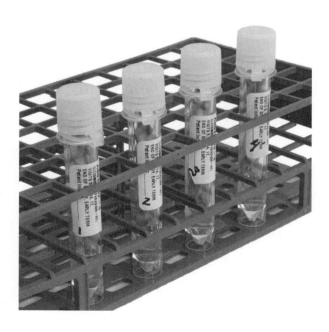

7. _____

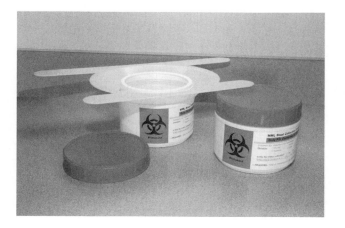

8. _____

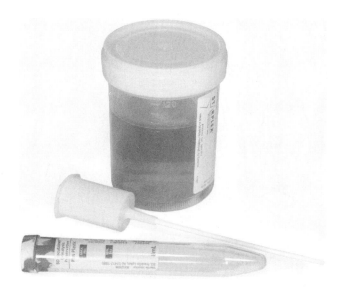

9. _____

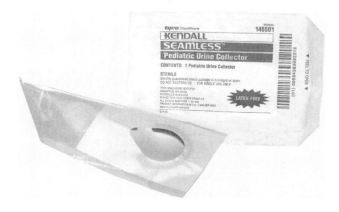

10. _____

LABELING EXERCISE 13-2: BODY FLUIDS

Identify the type of fluid that comes from each numbered area of the body sections illustrated below. Write the name of the fluid on the corresponding line.

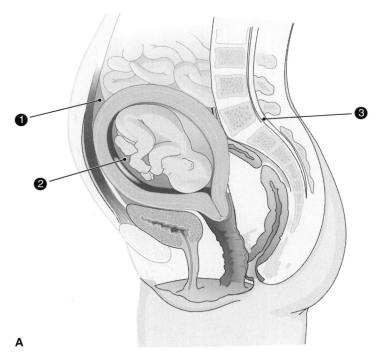

A

1. _____   3. _____

2. _____

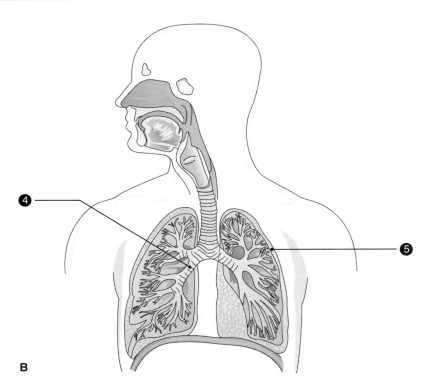

B

4. _____   5. _____

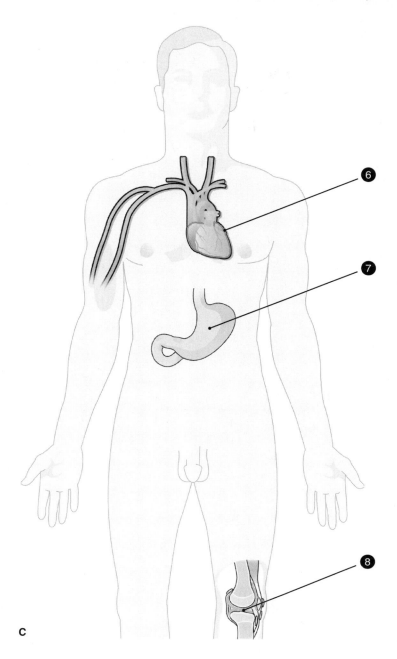

c

6. _____   8. _____

7. _____

Knowledge Drills

KNOWLEDGE DRILL 13-1: CAUTION AND KEY POINT RECOGNITION

The following sentences are taken from "CAUTION and KEY POINT" statements found throughout Chapter 13 in the TEXTBOOK. Using the TEXTBOOK, fill in the blanks with the missing information.

1. Phlebotomists are often asked to (A) _____ specimens to the (B) _____ that have been

   (C) _____ by other healthcare personnel. It is important for the phlebotomist to verify proper

   (D) _____ before (E) _____ a specimen for transport.

2. If (A) _____ specimens are not (B) _____ promptly, or preserved, (C) _____

   (D) _____ can change. For example, (E) _____ elements (F) _____, bilirubin

   breaks down to (G) _____, and bacteria multiply, leading to erroneous test results.

3. Urine specimens for (A) _____ and other (B) _____ tests should be transported to the

   lab and processed (C) _____. If a delay in transportation or processing is unavoidable the specimen

   should be (D) _____ or (E) _____.

4. A (A) _____ specimen should not be collected in a (B) _____ unless it is one specifi-

   cally designed for specimen collection. Regular (C) _____ often contain (D) _____

   (substances that (E) _____ (F) _____) that invalidate test results.

5. The patient must (A) _____ (B) _____ material from (C) _____ in the

   (D) _____ tract and not simply (E) _____ into the container.

6. _____ urine specimen collection instructions for patients must be accompanied by

   (B) _____ instructions, preferably with (C) _____. In outpatient areas, (D) _____

   instructions are often posted on the wall in the (E) _____ designated for patient urine collections.

7. A urine (A) _____ (B) _____ test also requires collection of a (C) _____

   creatinine specimen, which is ideally collected at the (D) _____ of urine collection. (i.e.,

   (E) _____ hours into urine collection).

8. The (A) _____ that causes TB (*Mycobacterium tuberculosis*) is often referred to as an

   (B) _____ - _____ (C) _____ (_____) because it resists decolorizing by acid after

   it has been stained. Likewise, the (D) _____ test for TB is often called an (E) _____

   culture, and the slide made from sputum is called an (F) _____ smear.

9. If a (A) _____ has been added to a urine collection container, patients must be

   (B) _____ not to (C) _____ directly into the container, to avoid being

   (D) _____ with the preservative.

10. A spinal tap is performed in the (A) _____ (B) _____ region of the spine. The spinal

    cord (C) _____ near the first or second lumbar vertebrae. To avoid (D) _____ to the

    spinal cord, the (E) _____ used to withdraw the CSF is inserted (F) _____ the third and

    fourth or the fourth and fifth lumbar vertebrae, well (G) _____ where the spinal cord ends.

KNOWLEDGE DRILL 13-2: SCRAMBLED WORDS

Unscramble the following words using the hints given in parenthesis and the letters that have been placed in the correct boxes. Finish writing the correct spelling of the scrambled word in the corresponding boxes.

1. tonimica (fluid surrounding a fetus)

		n			i	

2. spiboy (take a tissue sample)

b					

3. scoplebarneri (relating to the brain and spinal cord)

	e			r	o					

4. trueluc (grow microbes)

		l		u		

5. scirtag (relating to the stomach)

					i	c

6. sademtirm (in the middle of urination)

	i						a	

7. lucoct (hidden)

		c			

8. ispartaes (they live off other organisms)

			a					s

9. enoptralie (relating to the abdominal cavity)

	e		i					l

10. vistysintie (microbe susceptibility)

		n				i	v		

11. visonlay (of the joints)

s				v			

12. dovedi (urinated naturally)

				e	d

KNOWLEDGE DRILL 13-3: TRUE/FALSE ACTIVITY

The following statements are all false. Circle the one or two words that make the statement false and write the correct word(s) that would make the statement true in the space provided.

1. When asked to transport specimens to the lab, the phlebotomist should verify the proper billing information before accepting the specimen for transport.

2. In asking an outpatient for a urine specimen, the phlebotomist must be able to explain urine collection procedures without showing the patient.

3. The best time to begin a 24-hour collection is when the patient eats in the morning.

4. Semen specimens are collected in sterile or chemically clean containers and must be kept refrigerated and protected from the light, and delivered to the lab immediately.

5. For buccal swabs, the phlebotomist collects the sample by gently massaging the mouth on the inside of the gums with a special swab.

6. To prepare for the hydrogen breath test, the patient must not have taken antibiotics for at least 2 weeks before the test and must avoid certain foods for 24 hours prior to the test.

7. Patients are instructed, when collecting an FOBT, to follow a glucose-free diet for 3 days prior to the test.

8. A throat culture is typically collected using a special kit containing a sterile polyester-tipped swab in a covered petri dish containing transport medium.

9. Saliva specimens are sometimes collected in the diagnosis or monitoring of lower respiratory tract infections.

10. HCG may also appear in the urine of patients with diabetes or tumors of the ovaries or testes.

11. If urine samples/specimens are not tested promptly, urine components like bacteria die, leading to erroneous test results.

12. If a culture and sensitivity is ordered on a urine specimen, the container must be opaque.

KNOWLEDGE DRILL 13-4: RATIONALE FOR CLEAN-CATCH URINE PROCEDURE

Match each of the following rationales to the steps of the *Clean-Catch Urine Collection Procedure for Women* (Text Procedure 13-2) listed below. Place the appropriate letter in the Rationale column next to the step. (Rationales may be used more than once.)

Rationale

A. Aids in infection control

B. Aids in infection control and helps avoid contamination of the site while cleaning

C. Allows proper cleaning of the area

D. Helps ensure thorough cleaning by using fresh wipes for each area in a way that carries bacteria away from the urethral opening

E. Helps ensure sterility of the specimen, and that a sufficient amount of urine to perform the test is collected

F. Facilitates cleaning and downward flow of urine

G. Follow facility protocol

H. Disposes of excess urine

I. Helps maintain site antisepsis while initial urination helps wash away antiseptic residue and any microbes remaining in the urinary opening

J. Helps ensure the lid and container will remain sterile for accurate interpretation of results

K. Helps maintain sterility of the specimen

Steps   Rationale

1. Wash hands thoroughly   _____

2. Remove the lid of the container, being careful not to touch the inside of the cover or the container   _____

3. Stand in a squatting position over the toilet   _____

4. Separate the folds of skin around the urinary opening   _____

5. Cleanse the area on either side and around the opening with the special wipes, using a fresh wipe for each area and wiping from front to back. Discard used wipes in the trash   _____

6. While keeping the skin folds separated, void into the toilet for a few seconds   _____

7. Touching only the outside of the container and without letting it touch the genital area, bring the urine container into the urine stream until a sufficient amount of urine (30–100 mL) is collected   _____

8. Void any additional urine into the toilet   _____

9. Cover the specimen with the lid provided, touching only the *outside* surfaces of the lid and container   _____

10. Clean any urine on the outside of the container with an antiseptic wipe   _____

11. Wash hands   _____

12. Hand specimen to phlebotomist or place it where instructed if already labeled   _____

Skills Drills

SKILLS DRILL 13-1: REQUISITION ACTIVITY

The list of tests to choose from a laboratory requisition includes the nonblood tests listed below. Write the meaning of the test abbreviation (or NA if not abbreviated) and the type of specimen required on the corresponding line.

Test	Abbreviation Meaning	Type of Specimen
1. AFB	_____	_____
2. C. diff	_____	_____
3. CSF analysis	_____	_____
4. Carbon 13-urea	_____	_____
5. Diphtheria culture	_____	_____
6. Guaiac	_____	_____
7. HCG	_____	_____
8. L/S ratio	_____	_____
9. Male fertility studies	_____	_____
10. O&P	_____	_____
11. Rapid strep	_____	_____
12. TB culture	_____	_____
13. UA C&S	_____	_____

SKILLS DRILL 13-2: WORD BUILDING

Divide each word below into all of its elements (parts); prefix (P), word root (WR), combining vowel (CV), and suffix (S). Write the word part and its definition on the corresponding lines. Write the general meaning of the word in the space provided. If the word does not have a particular element, write NA (not applicable) in its place.

Example: gastric

Elements ___NA___ / ___gastr___ / ___NA___ / ___ic___
          P   WR   CV   S

Definitions ___NA___ / ___stomach___ / ___NA___ / ___pertaining___

Meaning: pertaining to the stomach

1. cerebrospinal

   Elements _____ / _____ / _____ / _____ / _____
             P   WR   CV   WR   S

   Definition _____ / _____ / _____ / _____

   Meaning:

2. cytology

   Elements _____ / _____ / _____ / _____
             P   WR   CV   S

   Definition _____ / _____ / _____ / _____

   Meaning:

3. hemolytic

Elements   _____ /_____ /_____ /_____ /_____

                             P   WR   CV   WR   S

Definition   _____ /_____ /_____ /_____ /_____

Meaning:

4. meningitis

Elements   _____ /_____ /_____ /_____

                             P   WR   CV   S

Definition   _____ /_____ /_____ /_____

Meaning:

5. nasopharyngitis

Elements   _____ /_____ /_____ /_____ /_____

                             P   WR   CV   WR   S

Definition   _____ /_____ /_____ /_____ /_____

Meaning:

6. pericardial

Elements   _____ /_____ /_____ /_____

                             P   WR   CV   S

Definition   _____ /_____ /_____ /_____

Meaning:

SKILLS DRILL 13-3: 24-HOUR URINE COLLECTION PROCEDURE (Text Procedure 13-1)

Fill in the blanks with the missing information.

Steps

1. Void into toilet as usual upon awakening.

2. Note the (C) _____ and _____ on the specimen label, place it on the container, and begin timing.

3. Collect all urine voided for the next 24 hours.

4. (G) _____ the specimen throughout the collection period if required.

   Note: Specimens can be kept cool in a refrigerator, or in a disposable ice chest placed in the bath tub, for example.

5. When a bowel movement is anticipated, collect the urine specimen (I) _____, not (J) _____ it.

Explanation/Rationale

Removes all urine from the previous time period and ensures that the bladder is (A) _____ when (B)_____ starts.

Verifies the date, timing, and patient (D) _____ information of the specimen for the laboratory.

Ensures results are based on the (E) _____ (F) _____ of urine produced in 24 hours.

Preserves analyte (H) _____.

Prevents (K) _____ contamination of the specimen.

6. Drink a normal amount of (L) _____ unless instructed to do otherwise.

7. Void one last time at the end of the 24 hours and add it to the collection container.

Prevents (M) _____ and facilitates specimen collection.

Ensures the (N) _____ volume of urine (O) _____ in the 24-hour period is collected.

Note: The morning specimen is typically the largest by (P) _____, the most (Q) _____, and an important part of the 24-hour urine collection.

8. Seal the container, place it in a portable cooler, unless instructed otherwise, and transport it to the laboratory (R) _____.

Helps protect the (S) _____ of the specimen.

SKILLS DRILL 13-4: THROAT CULTURE SPECIMEN COLLECTION PROCEDURE HIGHLIGHT SUMMARIES (Text Procedure 13-4)

The following are summaries of *Throat Culture Specimen Collection Procedure* highlights. Fill in the blanks with the missing information.

1. The phlebotomist may wish to wear a (A) _____ and goggles because throat culture collection will often cause the patient to have a gag reflex or to (B) _____.

2. Open container and remove swab in an (C) _____ manner because (D) _____ of the swab must be maintained for accurate (E) _____ of results.

3. Stand back or to the (F) _____ of the patient to help avoid contact with (G) _____ if the patient coughs.

4. Direct light onto the back of the throat using a small flashlight or other light source to illuminate areas of (H) _____, ulceration, (I) _____, or capsule formation.

5. Depress the tongue with a tongue depressor to help avoid touching other areas of the mouth and (J) _____ the sample during collection.

6. Saying "ah" raises the (K) _____ (soft tissue hanging from the back of the throat) out of the way.

7. Swab both (L) _____, tonsillar crypts (crevasses), the back of the throat, and any areas of ulceration, exudation, or inflammation, being careful not to touch the swab to the lips, (M) _____, or uvula.

8. Being careful not to touch the (N) _____ avoids a (O) _____ reflex.

9. Maintain (P) _____ (Q) _____ position while removing the swab to prevent the tongue from contaminating the swab.

10. Place the swab back in the transport tube, (R) _____ in (S) _____, and secure cover to keep the (T) _____ alive until they can be cultured in the laboratory.

Crossword

ACROSS

1. Urine sample collection method (two words)
6. _____ chloride test
7. Grow microbes on nutrient media
8. Aspirated from the bone
9. Urine screening to detect these substances
11. Coughed up from deep in the lungs
12. Hormone in urine after conception (abbrev.)
15. Test on urine sample
17. Normal antigen found in amniotic fluid (abbrev.)
19. Most frequently analyzed nonblood fluid
20. _____ syndrome
21. A sterile polyester-tipped collection device
22. Hidden blood in stool
23. _____ and parasites
26. Related to the lung
27. Fluid secreted from glands in the mouth
29. Urinalysis (abbrev.)
31. Synovial fluid found in this cavity
33. Urine specimen that requires watching the clock
35. Amniotic test indicating fetal lung maturity (abbrev.)
36. Sperm-containing fluid
37. Fluid surrounding a fetus in the uterus

DOWN

1. Means study of cells
2. Insert a collection tube through the urethra
3. Person who performs chemistry tests
4. Pertaining to the stomach
5. Serum-like fluid
6. Another name for feces
7. Fluid around brain and spinal cord (abbrev.; plural)
10. Throat culture to diagnosis this bacteria
13. Test for hidden blood in feces
14. Urine specimen collected at any time
15. Urinary tract infection (abbrev.)
16. Viscous fluid found in joint cavity
18. Cells inside of the cheek
24. Type of steroids used to enhance athletic ability
25. Liquid substances produced by the body
26. *Helicobacter* _____
28. To urinate
30. Prescribed course of eating
32. To examine
34. Analysis using buccal cells from inside the cheek

Chapter Review Questions

1. When accepting a specimen for transport to the lab from a nursing unit it is important to verify
   a. Billing code information
   b. Name of nurse requesting transport
   c. Patient identification information
   d. Physician requesting the test

2. Which of the following can be detected by chemical analysis of a urine specimen?
   a. Clarity
   b. Crystals
   c. Glucose
   d. All of the above

3. Sputum specimens are used to detect
   a. Cystic fibrosis
   b. Pregnancy
   c. Recent drug use
   d. Tuberculosis

4. This test is used to detect *Helicobacter pylori*
   a. AFB
   b. C-UBT
   c. Guaiac
   d. NP culture

5. Synovial fluid is aspirated from the
   a. Heart
   b. Lungs
   c. Joints
   d. Stomach

6. Pilocarpine is used in this test procedure
   a. Bone marrow biopsy
   b. Gastric analysis
   c. CSF collection
   d. Sweat chloride

7. Urine cytology studies can be performed to detect
   a. Alpha-fetoprotein
   b. Cytomegalovirus
   c. Infertility
   d. Meningitis

8. The specimen for this test requires stat handling and is typically collected by a physician in three or four sterile tubes.
   a. CSF analysis
   b. Gastric analysis
   c. Nasopharyngeal culture
   d. Suprapubic urine specimen

9. This test requires a 24-hour urine specimen.
   a. Creatinine clearance
   b. Glucose tolerance
   c. HCG detection
   d. Urine cytology

10. Which of the following would most likely lead to recollection of a drug screening specimen?
    a. pH is too low
    b. pH is too high
    c. SG is too low
    d. All of the above

11. A urine pregnancy test detects the presence of
    a. AFP
    b. DNA
    c. HCG
    d. UTI

12. This type of sample can show evidence of long-term drug use.
    a. Breath
    b. Feces
    c. Hair
    d. Saliva

13. Which of the following urine specimens will normally have the highest specific gravity?
    a. First morning
    b. Midstream
    c. Random
    d. 24-hour

14. A urine sensitivity test
    a. Detects inflammatory disorders
    b. Exposes antibiotic susceptibility
    c. Identifies a microorganism
    d. Screens for illegal drug use

15. Bone marrow samples are typically evaluated in
    a. Chemistry and microbiology
    b. Coagulation and blood bank
    c. Hematology and histology
    d. Serology and immunology

16. Problems in fetal development can be detected by studies on this fluid.
    a. Amniotic
    b. Gastric
    c. Spinal
    d. Synovial

17. A less invasive way than venipuncture to collect a specimen for DNA analysis is by:
    a. buccal swab
    b. NP swab
    c. sweat swab
    d. throat swab

18. Which of the following tests is used to monitor insulin therapy?
    a. 2-hour PP
    b. C-urea
    c. FOBT
    d. Sputum

19. When screening a patient's urine for drugs, which drug result is not quantitatively reliable?
    a. Alcohol
    b. Amphetamines
    c. Cannabinoids
    d. Methadone

20. When collecting spinal fluid for testing, why is the puncture performed in the lower lumbar region of the spinal column:
    a. the area is easier to access
    b. there is more fluid there
    c. to avoid spinal cord injury
    d. to insure blood-free fluid

Case Studies

Case Study 13-1: CSF Specimen Handling

A nurse delivered three vials of CSF to the lab. A phlebotomist newly trained in specimen processing accepted the specimens from the nurse. The phlebotomist had never received CSF specimens before and was not sure what to do with them. She was extremely busy and her supervisor was at lunch, so she set the vials aside, intending to ask her supervisor what to do with them upon her return from lunch. The supervisor got called to an emergency meeting and did not return for several hours. The phlebotomist was so busy she completely forgot about the CSF specimens until the physician called for the results on them. When he found out the specimens had not been tested he was furious. The specimens had to be recollected and the phlebotomist almost lost her job.

QUESTIONS

1. How could this incident have been prevented?

2. Why did the specimens have to be recollected?

3. How is a CSF specimen collected?

Case Study 13-2: Urine C&S Specimen Collection

Luann recently received on-the-job phlebotomy training. Today was the first day she had been allowed to work alone. It was a busy day and patients were starting to stack up in the waiting area. One elderly woman needed a blood test and a urine C&S. Luann was good at drawing blood and liked doing it. She hated to instruct patients in urine collection, however. She drew the blood specimen, quickly bandaged the patient and handed her a labeled urine collection container and several antiseptic wipes. She asked the patient if she had ever given a urine specimen for a culture before and when the patient said "Yes," she showed her where the restroom was, and told her that she should put the specimen on the counter when she was finished and then she could leave. She then called another patient in for a blood draw. The elderly woman came out of the rest room, set the specimen on the counter as she had been told and left. Later that day when things quieted down, Luann discovered that the patient had placed the antiseptic wipes in the urine container with the specimen. She was mad that the woman could be so foolish and also that she would have to call her and request that the woman return to the lab and submit a new specimen.

QUESTIONS

1. Why would the patient make such a mistake if she had submitted a urine specimen before?

2. What should Luann have done that would have prevented the problem with the specimen?

Case Study 13-3: AFB Culture

It was Friday morning in the small rural hospital, Gerry, the phlebotomist, had just finished his usual morning draws when the nurse handed him an order for an AFB culture and directed him to the patient who was in isolation. The phlebotomist had not seen this order before and asked the nurse if someone else could do it. The nurse said it needed to be done that morning and because they were short staffed he needed to advise the patient on how to collect the specimen. Before dressing to enter the room, he called his supervisor and was told to bring the request to the tech in the micro laboratory. He was relieved and quickly left the floor.

QUESTIONS

1. What does AFB mean?

2. What disease do they think the patient has?

3. What type of specimen would be collected and how should it be done?

Chapter 14

Arterial Puncture Procedures

Objectives

Study the information in your TEXTBOOK that corresponds to each objective to prepare yourself for the activities in this chapter.

1 Demonstrate knowledge of practices, terminology, hazards, and complications related to arterial blood collection, and identify and analyze arterial puncture sites according to site selection criteria and the advantages and disadvantages of each site.

2 Describe arterial blood gas (ABG) procedure including patient assessment and preparation, equipment and supplies, and commonly measured ABG parameters.

3 Perform the modified Allen Test; explain how to interpret results, and describe what to do based upon the results.

Matching

Use choices only once unless otherwise indicated.

MATCHING 14-1: KEY TERMS AND DESCRIPTIONS

Match each key term with the *best* description.

Key Terms (1–12)

1. _____ Abducted
2. _____ ABGs
3. _____ Allen test
4. _____ Arteriospasm
5. _____ Brachial artery
6. _____ Collateral circulation
7. _____ Femoral artery
8. _____ FiO$_2$
9. _____ L/M
10. _____ Radial artery
11. _____ Steady state
12. _____ Ulnar artery

Descriptions

A. Area is supplied with blood from more than one artery
B. Artery located in the antecubital fossa near the insertion of the biceps muscle
C. Artery located in the groin, lateral to the pubic bone
D. Artery located on the little-finger side of the wrist
E. Artery located on the thumb side of the wrist
F. Fraction of inspired oxygen, as in oxygen therapy
G. L/min, as in oxygen therapy
H. Out to the side, away from the body
I. Reflex or involuntary contraction of an artery
J. Stable condition with no exercise, suctioning, or respirator changes for 20 to 30 minutes
K. Test performed to assess collateral circulation before arterial puncture
L. Test used to assess a patient's oxygenation, ventilation, and acid–base balance

MATCHING 14-2: ARTERIES AND ADVANTAGES AND DISADVANTAGES

Match the arteries to the advantages and disadvantages associated with performing arterial punctures on them. Some advantages and disadvantages may have more than one choice.

Arteries
A. Radial
B. Brachial
C. Femoral

Advantages

1. _____ easy to compress after puncture
2. _____ fairly close to the surface of the skin
3. _____ has the best collateral circulation
4. _____ large and easy to palpate
5. _____ less chance of hematoma formation
6. _____ may be only choice during low cardiac output
7. _____ no major nerves or veins immediately adjacent
8. _____ preferred for collection of large volumes of blood

Disadvantages

1. _____ deeply located
2. _____ hardest to locate during low cardiac output
3. _____ increased chance of dislodging plaque
4. _____ increased risk of hematoma formation
5. _____ increased risk of infection
6. _____ lies close to a major vein
7. _____ lies close to the median nerve
8. _____ no underlying ligaments or bone
9. _____ poor collateral circulation
10. _____ small size requires more skill to puncture

Labeling Exercises

LABELING EXERCISE 14-1: ARM AND LEG ARTERIES (Figs. 14-2 and 14-3)

Identify each artery of the arm and leg identified by the numbered arrows and write the name on the corresponding numbered line below.

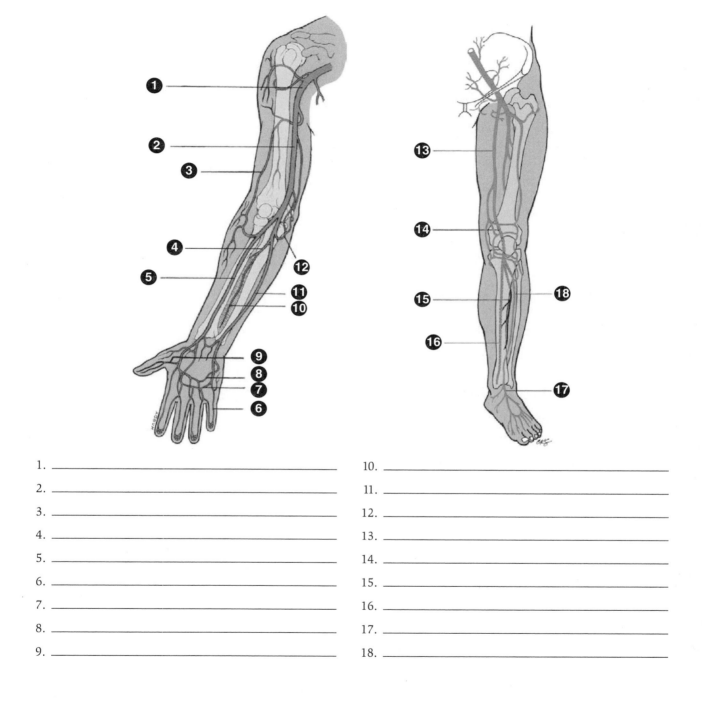

1. _____
2. _____
3. _____
4. _____
5. _____
6. _____
7. _____
8. _____
9. _____

10. _____
11. _____
12. _____
13. _____
14. _____
15. _____
16. _____
17. _____
18. _____

LABELING EXERCISE 14-2: ARTERIAL PUNCTURE SITES

Draw X's on the approximate sites on the arm where arterial puncture is performed. Write "1" next to the X on the site that is the first choice for arterial puncture. Write the name of the first choice artery on line 1 below. Write the name of the other artery on line 2.

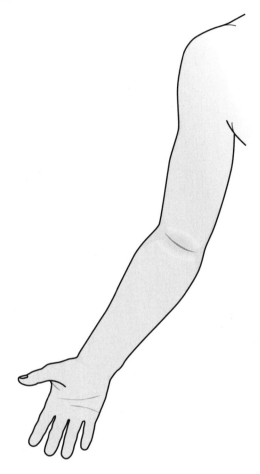

1. _____

2. _____

Knowledge Drills

KNOWLEDGE DRILL 14-1: CAUTION AND KEY POINT RECOGNITION

The following sentences are "CAUTION and KEY POINT" statements found throughout Chapter 14 in the TEXTBOOK. Using the TEXTBOOK, fill in the blanks with the missing information.

1. *Never* select a site in a limb with an (A) _____ or (B) _____. It is a patient's lifeline

    for (C) _____ and should not be disturbed; also, venous and arterial blood (D) _____

    _____ at the site.

2. *Never* use the (A) _____ to (B) _____, as it has a (C) _____ that can be

    misleading.

3. *Do not* (A) _____. (B) _____ is painful and can cause (C) _____ or

    (D) _____ formation, or damage the artery.

4. *Never* allow the patient to (A) _____ the (B) _____. A patient may not

    (C) _____ it firmly enough. In addition, *do not* replace use of (D) _____ _____

    for the required length of time with the application of a pressure bandage.

5. *Never* leave the patient if the site is still (A) _____. If (B) _____ _____

    _____ _____ within a reasonable time, notify the patient's (C) _____ or

    (D) _____ of the problem.

6. According to CLSI, the (A) _____ artery in children, especially infants, is not commonly used

    because it is (B) _____ to (C) _____ and lacks (D) _____ _____.

KNOWLEDGE DRILL 14-2: SCRAMBLED WORDS

Unscramble the following words using the hints given in parenthesis and the letters that have been placed in the correct boxes. Finish writing the correct spelling of the scrambled word in the corresponding box.

1. cudadebt (arm position for ABG collection)

	b				t		

2. dalira (artery released first in an Allen test)

		d			

3. egxony (analyte measured by an ABG test)

	x				

4. eydats (patient state for accurate ABGs)

s					

5. fiddemoi (changed from the original)

		d			e	

6. nivetonliat (air entering and leaving the lungs)

			t		l	a				

7. oltraclela (circulation requirement for arterial puncture)

		l	l						

8. slavogava (relating to a reaction by a particular nerve)

		s				g		

9. smearpotrisa (vessel reaction to arterial puncture)

a						o		a		

10. tencheasti (a substance that dulls pain)

							t		c	

11. traleria (specimen required for ABGs)

		t				a		

12. vanigtee (Allen test result that means "choose another site")

n		g					

KNOWLEDGE DRILL 14-3: TRUE/FALSE ACTIVITY

The following statements are all false. Circle the one or two words that make the statement false and write the correct word(s) that would make the statement true in the space provided.

1. The modified Allen test checks for the presence of collateral circulation to the hand via the radial artery.

_____

2. Arterial puncture is typically less painful than venipuncture. _____

3. Color is, in fact, a reliable indicator of successful arterial puncture. _____

4. The proper angle of needle insertion for femoral artery puncture is 45 degrees. _____

5. Steady state for ABG collection, means the patient has had no food. _____

6. Specimens for electrolyte testing in addition to arterial blood gas (ABG) analysis should be transported on ice.

_____

7. After performing arterial puncture, the respiration is checked distal to ensure no damage has occurred during

the draw. _____

8. Injury to the intima, or inner wall of the artery, can lead to a hematoma. _____

9. Phlebitis is a complication associated with arterial puncture. _____

10. The femoral artery is the second choice for arterial puncture for ABGs. _____

KNOWLEDGE DRILL 14-4: HAZARDS AND COMPLICATIONS OF ARTERIAL PUNCTURE

List eight hazards or complications of arterial puncture.

1. _____
2. _____
3. _____
4. _____
5. _____
6. _____
7. _____
8. _____

KNOWLEDGE DRILL 14-5: SAMPLING ERRORS

List seven sampling errors associated with ABG collection.

1. _____
2. _____
3. _____
4. _____
5. _____
6. _____
7. _____

KNOWLEDGE DRILL 14-6: CRITERIA FOR SPECIMEN REJECTION

List eight criteria for specimen rejection and state how you would prevent such a rejection from happening.

Rejection Criteria	Prevention Tactic
1. _____	_____
	_____
2. _____	_____
	_____
3. _____	_____
	_____
4. _____	_____
	_____
5. _____	_____
	_____
6. _____	_____
	_____
7. _____	_____
	_____
8. _____	_____

KNOWLEDGE DRILL 14-7: COMMONLY MEASURED ABG ANALYTES (Table 14-1)

Fill in the blanks with the missing information.

Analyte	Normal Range	Description
PH	(A) _____	A measure of the (B) _____ or (C) _____ of the blood; used to identify a condition such as acidosis or alkalosis.
(D) _____	80–100 mm Hg	Partial pressure of (E) _____ in arterial blood. A measure of how much (F) _____ is dissolved in the blood. Indicates if (G) _____ is adequate. Decreased (H) _____ levels in the blood increase the respiration rate and vice versa.
PaCO$_2$	35–45 (I) _____	Partial pressure of (J) _____ _____ in arterial blood. A measure of how much (K) _____ _____ is dissolved in the blood. Evaluates (L) _____ function. Increased CO$_2$ levels in the blood increase the (M) _____ rate and vice versa. *Respiratory* disturbances alter PaCO$_2$ levels.
(N) _____	22–26 mEq/L	(O) _____. A measure of the amount of (P) _____ in the blood. Evaluates the bicarbonate buffer system of the kidneys. *Metabolic* and *respiratory* disturbances alter HCO$_3$ levels.
O$_2$ saturation	97%–100%	Oxygen saturation. The percent of (Q) _____ bound to (R) _____. Determines if (S) _____ is carrying the amount of (T) _____ it is capable of carrying.
Base excess (or deficit)	(−2)–(+2) mEq/L	A calculation of the (U) _____ part of acid–base balance based on the PCO$_2$, HCO$_3$, and hemoglobin.

Skills Drills

SKILLS DRILL 14-1: REQUISITION ACTIVITY

A physician sends a patient to a hospital outpatient laboratory with the stat order shown below.

John Chursdt, MD
2011 Happy Street
Suite 9
Any Town USA

Lic.# 000000

Name _Jane Doe_ _____ Age _66_ _____

Address _____ Date _Sept. 19, 2015_ _____

℞

ABGs & L'Ytes

Patient has hx COPD
WBC drawn yesterday elevated

Signature _JChursdt, MD_ _____

---

1. What effect does a high WBC have on ABGs? _____

_____

_____

_____

2. How many draws will it take to collect specimens for all of the ordered tests? _____

_____

_____

_____

3. What type of syringe should be used to collect the ABG specimen? _____

_____

4. How should the specimen(s) be transported? _____

_____

SKILLS DRILL 14-2: WORD BUILDING

Divide each word into all of its elements (parts): prefix (P), word root (WR), combining vowel (CV), and suffix (S). Write the word part and its definition on the corresponding lines. Write the general meaning of the word in the space provided. If the word does not have a particular element, write NA (not applicable) in its place.

Example: asepsis

Elements _____*a*_____ /_____*sep*_____ /_____ /_____*sis*_____
                    P   WR   CV   S

Definitions ___*without*___ /_*pathogenic organisms*_ /_____ /___*condition of*___

Meaning: condition of being without pathogenic organisms

1. Acidosis

   Elements _____ /_____ /_____ /_____
                      P   WR   CV   S

   Definitions _____ /_____ /_____ /_____

   Meaning:

2. Anaerobic

   Elements _____ /_____ /_____ /_____
                      P   WR   CV   S

   Definitions _____ /_____ /_____ /_____

   Meaning:

3. Anesthetic

   Elements _____ /_____ /_____ /_____
                      P   WR   CV   S

   Definitions _____ /_____ /_____ /_____

   Meaning:

4. Arteriospasm

   Elements _____ /_____ /_____ /_____
                      P   WR   CV   S

   Definitions _____ /_____ /_____ /_____

   Meaning:

5. Brachial

   Elements _____ /_____ /_____ /_____
                      P   WR   CV   S

   Definitions _____ /_____ /_____ /_____

   Meaning:

6. Femoral

   Elements _____ /_____ /_____ /_____
                      P   WR   CV   S

   Definitions _____ /_____ /_____ /_____

   Meaning:

7. Hypodermic

   Elements _____ /_____ /_____ /_____
                      P   WR   CV   S

   Definitions _____ /_____ /_____ /_____

   Meaning:

8. Radial

Elements   _____ / _____ / _____ / _____
                    P   WR   CV   S

Definitions   _____ / _____ / _____ / _____

Meaning:

SKILLS DRILL 14-3: MODIFIED ALLEN TEST PROCEDURE (Procedure 14-1)

Fill in the blanks with the missing information.

Step

1. Have the patient make a tight fist.

2. Use the middle and index fingers of both hands to apply pressure to the patient's wrist, compressing both the (C) _____ and (D) _____ arteries at the same time.

3. While maintaining pressure, have the patient open the hand slowly. It should appear (G) _____ or drained of color.

4. Lower the patient's hand and release pressure on the (L) _____ artery only.

5. Assess results:

   Positive Allen test result: The hand (P) _____ _____ or returns to normal color within 15 seconds.

   Negative Allen test result: The hand (S) _____ _____ _____ _____ or return to normal color

6. Record the results on the (W). _____.

Explanation/Rationale

A tight fist partially blocks (A) _____ _____, causing temporary (B) _____ until the hand is opened.

Pressure over both arteries is needed to (E) _____ blood flow, which is required to be able to assess (F) _____ _____ when pressure is released.

(H) _____ appearance of the hand verifies temporary blockage of both arteries. Note: The patient must not (I) _____ the fingers when opening the hand, as this can cause (J) _____ blood flow and (K) _____ of results.

The (M) _____ artery is released while the (N) _____ is still obstructed to determine if it will be able to provide blood flow should the (O) _____ artery be injured during ABG collection.

A positive test result indicates return of blood to the hand via the (Q) _____ artery and the (R) _____ of collateral circulation. If the Allen test is positive, proceed with ABG collection. A negative test result indicates inability of the (T) _____ artery to adequately supply blood to the hand and therefore the (U) _____ of collateral circulation. If the Allen test result is negative, the (V) _____ artery should not be used and another site must be selected.

Verification that the Allen test was performed.

SKILLS DRILL 14-4: RADIAL ABG PROCEDURE (Procedure 14-3)

Fill in the blanks with the missing information.

Step

1. (A) _____ and accession test request.

2. Approach, identify, and prepare patient.

3. Check for sensitivities to latex and other substances.

4. Assess (F) _____ _____, verify collection requirements, and record required information.

5. (I) _____ hands and put on gloves.

6. Assess (K) _____ circulation.

7. Position arm, ask patient to (P) _____ wrist.

Explanation/Rationale

The requisition must be reviewed for completeness of information (see Chapter 8, "Venipuncture Procedure," step 1) and required collection (B) _____, such as oxygen delivery system, and (C) _____ or L/M.

Correct approach to the patient, identification, and preparation are essential (see Chapter 8, "Venipuncture Procedure," step 2). Preparing the patient by explaining the procedure in a calm and reassuring manner encourages cooperation and reduces apprehension. ((D) _____ due to anxiety, breath-holding, or crying can alter test results.)

Increasing numbers of individuals are allergic to latex, (E) _____, and other substances.

Required collection conditions must be met and must not have changed for (G) _____ prior to collection. Test results can be meaningless or misinterpreted and patient care compromised if they have not been met. The patient's temperature, respiratory rate, and FiO_2 affect blood gas (H) _____ and must be recorded along with other required information.

Proper hand hygiene plays a major role in (J) _____ _____, protecting the phlebotomist, patient, and others from contamination. Gloves provide a barrier to bloodborne pathogen exposure. Gloves may be put on at this point or later, depending on hospital protocol.

(L) _____ circulation must be verified by either the modified (M) _____ test, ultrasonic flow indicator, or both. Proceed if result is (N) _____; choose another site if (O) _____.

The arm should be (Q) _____ with the palm up and the wrist (R) _____ approximately 30 degrees to stretch and fix the soft tissues over the firm ligaments and bone. (Avoid (S) _____, as it can eliminate a palpable pulse.)

8. Locate the radial artery and clean the site.

The (T) _____ _____ is used to locate the radial pulse (U) _____ to the skin crease on the (V) _____ side of the wrist; palpate it to determine size, depth, and direction. An arterial site is typically cleaned with alcohol or another suitable antiseptic and must not be touched again until the phlebotomist is ready to access the artery.

9. Administer local (W) _____ (optional).

Document anesthetic application on the requisition (Procedure 14–2).

10. Prepare equipment and clean gloved nondominant finger.

Assemble ABG equipment and set the (X) _____ _____ to the proper fill level if applicable. Gloves must be put on at this point if this has not already been done, and the nondominant finger cleaned, so that it does not contaminate the site when relocating the pulse before needle entry.

11. Pick up equipment and uncap and inspect needle.

The syringe is held in the dominant hand as if holding a (Y) _____. The needle must be inspected for defects, and replaced if any are found.

12. Relocate radial artery and warn patient of (Z) _____ _____.

The artery is relocated by placing the nondominant index finger directly over the (AA) _____. The patient is warned to prevent a (BB) _____ _____ and asked to relax the wrist to help ensure a smooth needle entry.

13. Insert the needle at a 30- to 45-degree angle, slowly direct it toward the (CC) _____, and stop when a (DD) _____ of blood appears.

A needle inserted at a 30- to 45-degree angle 5 to 10 mm (EE) _____ to the finger that is over the pulse should contact the artery directly under that finger. When the artery is entered, a (FF) _____ of blood normally appears in the needle hub or syringe. Note: If a needle smaller than 23-gauge is used, it may be necessary to pull gently on the syringe plunger to obtain blood flow.

14. Allow the syringe to fill to the proper level.

Blood will normally fill the syringe under its own (GG) _____, which is an indication that the specimen is indeed arterial blood. (See exception in step 13.)

15. Place gauze, remove needle, activate safety feature, and (HH) _____ _____.

A clean, folded gauze square is placed over the site, so firm manual pressure can be applied by the (II) _____ immediately upon needle removal and for 3 to 5 minutes thereafter. The needle safety device must be activated as soon as possible in order to prevent an accidental needlestick.

16. Remove and discard syringe needle.

For safety reasons, the specimen must not be transported with the needle attached to the syringe. The needle must be removed and discarded in the sharps container with one hand while site pressure is applied with the other.

17. Expel (JJ) _____ _____, cap syringe, mix and label specimen.

(KK) _____ _____ in the specimen can affect test results and must be expelled per manufacturer's instructions. While still holding pressure, the specimen must be capped to maintain (LL) _____ conditions, mixed thoroughly by inversion or rotating to prevent clotting, labeled with required information, and, if applicable, placed in coolant to protect analytes from the effects of cellular metabolism.

18. Check patient's arm and apply bandage.

The site is checked for swelling or bruising after pressure has been applied for 3 to 5 minutes. If the site is warm and appears normal, pressure is applied for 2 more minutes, after which the (MM) _____ is checked (NN) _____ to the site to confirm normal blood flow. If pulse and site are normal, a pressure bandage is applied and the time at which it should be removed is noted. Note: If the pulse is weak or absent, the patient's nurse or physician must be notified immediately.

19. Dispose off used and contaminated materials, remove gloves, and sanitize hands.

Used and contaminated items must be disposed off per facility protocol. Gloves must be removed and hands sanitized as an (OO) _____ _____ _____.

20. Thank patient, and transport specimen to the laboratory (PP) _____.

Thanking the patient is courteous and professional behavior. Prompt delivery of the specimen to the laboratory protects specimen (QQ) _____.

Crossword

ACROSS

1. Involuntary arterial contraction
5. With air
7. Mass of blood in the tissue
9. Concerning palm of the hand
10. Type of microbe
11. ABG collection equipment
12. The preferred one for ABG is 22-gauge
13. Hit the artery, see a _____
14. Preferred point of entry
17. Allen test checks for _____ flow
18. Syringe part capped after collection (2 words)
21. Arterial blood gas (abbrev.)
23. Test for collateral flow
25. Contaminant of ABGs
26. ABG component measured
27. Possible Allen test result

DOWN

1. Without air
2. Another name for clot
3. Protective equipment (abbrev.)
4. First-choice ABG site
6. Second-choice AB site
7. Anticoagulant for ABGs
8. Abrupt loss of consciousness response
13. ABG site used by physicians
15. Lidocaine, for one
16. Artery in the wrist
19. Hold the ABG syringe like a _____
20. Unacceptable way to find an artery
22. PPEs for hands
23. 30- to 45-degree _____ for ABGs
24. Anesthetic used to _____ site

Chapter Review Questions

1. Which of the following personnel may be required to perform arterial puncture?
   - a. EMTs
   - b. MTs
   - c. Phlebotomists
   - d. All of the above

2. O_2 saturation measures the:
   - a. alkalinity of the blood plasma.
   - b. amount of oxygen dissolved in the plasma.
   - c. oxygen pressure in the lungs.
   - d. percent of oxygen bound to hemoglobin.

3. Which is the first-choice artery for ABG collection?
   - a. Brachial
   - b. Femoral
   - c. Radial
   - d. Ulnar

4. Which of the following is the most important criterion for selecting an artery for ABG collection provided that there is no other reason to avoid the site?
   - a. Collateral circulation
   - b. Depth of the artery
   - c. Dominance of the arm
   - d. Strength of the pulse

5. The anticoagulant used in ABG specimen collection is:
   - a. EDTA.
   - b. heparin.
   - c. potassium oxalate.
   - d. sodium citrate.

6. In addition to identification information, which of the following is typically documented before ABG specimen collection?
   - a. FiO_2 or L/M
   - b. History of smoking
   - c. Room temperature
   - d. All of the above

7. A phlebotomist must collect an ABG specimen when the patient is breathing room air. The patient has just been taken off the ventilator when the phlebotomist arrives. When can the phlebotomist draw the ABG specimen?
   - a. After 1 hour
   - b. Immediately
   - c. In 5 to 10 minutes
   - d. In 20 to 30 minutes

8. A phlebotomist has a request to collect an ABG specimen on a patient. The patient has a positive Allen test on the right arm. What should the phlebotomist do?
   - a. Collect the specimen by capillary puncture.
   - b. Collect the specimen from the right radial artery.
   - c. Collect the specimen from the right ulnar artery.
   - d. Perform the Allen test on the left arm.

9. Which of the following is an acceptable range of needle gauges for arterial puncture?
   - a. 16 to 21
   - b. 18 to 23
   - c. 20 to 25
   - d. 23 to 28

10. In performing radial artery puncture, the needle should enter the skin:
    - a. at the exact point where the pulse is felt.
    - b. distal to where the pulse is felt.
    - c. lateral to where the pulse is felt.
    - d. proximal to where the pulse is felt.

11. Normally, when the needle enters the artery:
    - a. a flash of blood appears in the syringe.
    - b. the syringe plunger starts to vibrate.
    - c. you may hear a soft swishing sound.
    - d. all of the above can happen.

12. An ABG specimen is most likely to be rejected if it:
    - a. arrives at the laboratory 20 minutes after collection.
    - b. contains only around 2 mL of blood.
    - c. is collected in a glass syringe.
    - d. is determined to be QNS.

13. Which of the following is the best way to tell that the specimen you are collecting is in fact arterial blood?
    - a. A flash of blood appeared in the syringe on needle entry.
    - b. Blood pulsed into the syringe under its own power.
    - c. The color of the blood is bright cherry-red.
    - d. There is no way to tell for certain.

14. A single routine arterial specimen for both ABG and electrolyte testing should be transported:
    - a. at room temperature.
    - b. green-top tube.
    - c. on ice.
    - d. STAT.

15. The risk of hematoma associated with arterial puncture is greatest if:
    - a. a large-diameter needle is used.
    - b. the patient is elderly.
    - c. the patient is on a blood thinner.
    - d. all of the above.

Case Studies

Case Study 14-1: Modified Allen Test and ABG Specimen Collection

A phlebotomist has a request to collect a STAT ABG specimen on a patient. He had collected an ABG specimen the night before from the same patient on the same arm, and since the patient had a positive modified Allen test then, he skips the Allen test now to save time. As he is preparing to insert the needle, the patient's nurse enters the room and tells him to stop. She tells him that the patient does not have adequate collateral circulation in that arm and he must not collect the specimen there.

QUESTIONS

1. What error did the phlebotomist make?
2. How could the error have been avoided?
3. What could have caused the change in collateral circulation?

Case Study 14-2: ABG Hazards and Complications

A phlebotomist had an order to collect STAT ABG and electrolyte specimens from a patient in the ICU. The patient was having difficulty breathing when the phlebotomist arrived. There was an IV in the patient's right arm, so the phlebotomist performed the Allen test on the left arm. The test result was positive, so the phlebotomist proceeded to collect the specimen from the radial artery of that arm. He had to redirect the needle several times before dark bluish-red blood finally pulsed into the syringe. When the syringe was filled to the proper level, he withdrew the needle and held pressure over the site. As he was attempting to cap the syringe, the cap dropped into the patient's bed covers, so the phlebotomist asked the patient to hold pressure while he retrieved it. Later, when he went to check the arm, a large hematoma had formed at the collection site. When he checked the patient's pulse below the collection site, it was so weak he could barely feel it.

QUESTIONS

1. What could have caused the weak pulse and what should the phlebotomist do about it?
2. What error did the phlebotomist make that contributed to hematoma formation?
3. What would cause the specimen to be bluish red?
4. How can the phlebotomist be certain that the specimen is arterial blood?

Case Study 14-3: Brachial Artery Puncture Problem

A phlebotomist is sent to collect an ABG specimen from a patient in the cardiac care unit (CCU). The patient has an IV in the right arm near the wrist and the left wrist has a rash. The phlebotomist has been trained to do brachial artery punctures, so he decides to use the brachial artery of the left arm. The physician has specifically requested that the specimen be drawn without the use of lidocaine. The phlebotomist verifies that all other patient conditions have been met and proceeds with specimen collection. As he inserts the needle the patient winces in apparent great pain and moves his arm. No blood flows so the phlebotomist cautions the patient to keep still and redirects the needle. The syringe then rapidly fills with blood and the phlebotomist completes the draw. The phlebotomist holds pressure and then applies a pressure bandage, finishes the paperwork, and returns to the laboratory with the specimen.

QUESTIONS

1. Why might the physician have purposely requested that the specimen be drawn without lidocaine?
2. What should the phlebotomist have done when the patient felt great pain?
3. What nerve lies near the brachial artery and may have caused the pain response?

Unit IV Crossword Exercise

ACROSS

3. Term for urine collected in the middle of urination
5. Determines compatibility for blood transfusion
7. Activated partial thromboplastin time (abbrev.)
11. With air
13. *Hyponatremia* means this substance in the blood is decreased
14. Test for collateral flow
16. Involuntary contraction of an artery
18. Ailment caused by microorganisms somewhere in the urinary tract
19. Machine used to spin blood tubes
22. O&P test detects these
23. Evacuated tube with separator gel (abbrev.)
24. Type of fluid that surrounds fetus in the uterus
26. Secret code that allows access to a computer system
29. Type of swab collected from inside of cheek
30. Computer key that sends data to the processor
31. Image on a computer screen that represents a program
32. Type of testing done on the Cholestech instrument
35. Networking device that routes and forwards information
38. Iontophoresis is used to stimulate production of this body fluid

DOWN

1. Inhibiting agent in BC bottles to inhibit microorganism growth (abbrev.)
2. Test used to diagnose problems of carbohydrate metabolism
4. Phrase intended to assist memory
6. Microorganisms or their toxins in the blood
8. Often called alternate-site testing
9. Another name for sorting and processing
10. Type of circulation in which more than one artery supplies blood to an area
12. Sets standards for laboratory medicine (abbrev.)
13. Immediately
15. _____ agglutinins (temp. sensitivity)
17. Point at which the needle will actually enter the skin
18. Analysis of urine (abbrev.)
20. Type of fluid collected from the stomach
21. Artery located at the thumb side of the wrist
25. Hidden
27. Brachial or radial
28. A buccal swab is used for this analysis
33. Tube used for separating plasma and free-flowing cells
34. Fed. agency offering 10 steps to urine drug collection.
36. Time it takes from collection to results (abbrev.)
37. Main processor memory (abbrev.)

RRW0515